Natural Birth
and the
Faith-Filled Mother

Lyra M. Camacho

Natural Birth and the Faith-Filled Mother

ISBN 978-0-6151-4531-0

Dedication

For those who know me, the following pages are a mere reflection of who I am as a woman, a wife, a mother, and a believer. I dedicate this book to all of you, and especially to those that follow:

To my late mother, Barbara H. Goodchild. She spent many years in the health and natural food industry and therefore sparked my ongoing interest. I am also forever indebted to her for leading me to salvation. She is greatly missed.

To my wonderful husband, Joel, and the three beautiful children that we share. It is my God-given career to be his wife and their mother and it has brought immeasurable happiness.

To two friends of mine, Megan and Melanie Dawn. They have led me to a deeper relationship with the Lord by helping me realize that the Old Testament is still useful and valid.

To a long-lost friend and mentor, Miss Terry. She is a mother figure to me and has shown great kindness over the years. She is truly a wise and faith-filled woman.

And ultimately, I dedicate this book to the Lord. I hope that He will use it to bless other faith-filled families as He has blessed mine.

Thank You All,
Lyra M. Camacho

Disclaimer

The information provided in this book is based on the author's research and personal experience, as well as the teachings of the Holy Bible. This book is sold with the understanding that the author is not a medical professional. The author is also not liable or responsible for any loss or damage caused directly or indirectly by the information in this book. If you choose to use the information provided in this book, which is your constitutional right, the author assumes no responsibility.

In addition, it is not the author's intent for this book to serve as a complete guide to pregnancy, birth, and parenting. It is the author's recommendation, and your responsibility, to thoroughly research the subject matter in order to make well-informed decisions. Childbirth is a serious event and should not be taken lightly.

Contents

Chapter 1

Infertility	3
A Bit of Faith	4
Miscarriage	9
My Baby Journal	15

Chapter 2

To Plan or Not To Plan?	21
Are You Pregnant?	23
When Are You Due?	25
Where to Deliver?	25
In-Hospital Birthing Centers	29
Freestanding Birthing Centers	30
Home-Birth Midwives	30
Unassisted Home-Births	31
Prenatal Care	32
Weight	32
Blood Pressure	33
Diet	33
Rest and Exercise	36
Baby's Movement	37
Daily Prayer	37
In Addition. . .	38
Prenatal Checklist	39

Chapter 3

Pregnancy: What to Expect   41
Common Pregnancy Complaints   44
Problems in Pregnancy   47
Spiritual Preparation   50
The Child Within   53
Your Baby's Development   53

Chapter 4

Birthing Supplies   57
Preparing for Labor   59
Labor and Delivery Comfort Measures   60
Doula Care   62
Preparing for Birth   63
Birth Preparation Exercises   64
Signs of Labor   65
      Potential Signs   65
      Preliminary Signs   66
      Positive Signs   67
The Labor and Delivery Process   68
Labor and Delivery: What to Expect   70
Your Newborn   72
Postpartum   73

Chapter 5

Breast-Feeding   75
Vaccinations   81
Diapering   83
Sleeping   85
Discipline   95
Entertainment   97
Schooling   98
To Work or Not To Work?   102

Chapter 6

The Lasting Pain of Childbirth   105

Traumatic Birth   116
Vaginal Birth After Cesarean   118

Chapter 7
A Healing Home-Birth   123
Overcoming Home-Birth Obstacles   133
Birth: A Closer Look   134

Chapter 8 (A Home-Birth Journal)
The First Trimester   143
The Second Trimester   157

Chapter 9 (A Home-Birth Journal)
The Third Trimester   165
The Labor and Delivery   176
Postpartum   183

Chapter 10
Poetry   185

Chapter 11 (Rh Negative Information)
My Story   205
What is Rh Negative?   207
Using Rhogam: The Risks   208
Not Using Rhogam: The Risks   208
Changing Rh Status   209
Preventing Sensitization   210
The Sensitized Mother   211
Lifestyle Regimen for the Rh Negative Mother   213
    Step 1: Detoxification   213
    Step 2: Health-Promoting Diet   214
    Step 3: Health-Promoting Lifestyle   215
    Step 4: Building and Purifying Blood   216
    Step 5: Gentle Birth   218

Chapter 12 (Prayers & Confessions)

Salvation 219

Infertility 221

Pregnancy 223

Threatened Miscarriage 224

Vaginal Birth After Cesarean 226

Rh Negative Mothers 227

Delivery 228

Baby Dedication 230

Final Thoughts 233

About the Author 235

Bibliography 237

Introduction

I am not a doctor, a midwife, or a certified professional of any kind. Instead, I am a faith-filled wife and mother with an unyielding passion for doing things naturally. And by *naturally*, I am referring to the way that our Creator intended.

Throughout my parenting journey, I have sadly discovered that most information on natural birth and parenting is laced with unnatural religion. Yet strangely, the most natural way of all is God's way. It isn't anything alternative or new-age. It is simply the way that things have been since the beginning of time. God is the Creator and there is nothing more God-honoring than doing things as He intended.

Chapter One

For many of us, having children comes naturally and easily. It takes nine months for the mere desire to conceive to result in a bundle of joy. It is as simple as boy meets girl; boy marries girl; boy and girl have a baby. But quite often, it isn't that simple.

Sometimes conception is difficult. Sometimes each month turns into an emotional whirlwind with not-so-promising results. And sometimes conception doesn't result in a baby at all. Instead, it results in the loss of a baby. But with God, it doesn't have to be that way.

Infertility

This book would not be complete without addressing a common issue among many God-fearing couples–infertility. It affects so many of us, and although modern medicine has a way of dealing with it, God's way is always better.

My husband and I dealt with infertility for the first four years of our marriage. I know firsthand about the monthly cycle of hope, anticipation, and heartbreak. And, as you'll see in the following article that I wrote, I also know firsthand what can be done with a bit of faith.

A Bit of Faith

For as long as I can remember, I have always wanted to be a mother–not the mother of one, but of many. And although life has brought about many aspirations, none were as great as my desire to have children.

My husband and I were married at the age of eighteen, and we wasted no time in trying to conceive. Each month carried the possibility of pregnancy, and I earnestly longed to see my dreams fulfilled.

Yet as promising as each month began, they all ended in disappointment. Soon the months turned into years, and I hid from the reality that I was too afraid to admit. What if we couldn't have children?

Many nights I'd cry myself to sleep. Infertility seemed more than I could bear, and the only peace I'd find was in the Lord. I knew that I wouldn't want to be a mother so wholeheartedly if I wasn't meant to be one. I also knew that with God, all things were possible.

A single doctor's visit confirmed my worst fear–we couldn't have children. Although I had known it all along in my heart, reality had officially spoken.

The news wasn't as life-shattering as I had imagined. Instead, it brought closure. I had been battling infertility for quite some time, but it was finally over. My desire to conceive wasn't over. No, not by far. But relying on human understanding had breathed its last.

Shortly after, I read the following verse. It was something that I had seen many times before, but on that day, it spoke to me.

Matthew 18:19-20 Again, I tell you that if two of you on earth agree about anything you ask for, it will be done for you by my Father in heaven. For where two or three come together in my name, there am I with them.

At that time in our marriage, my husband and I didn't

openly pray together. However, I knew that I needed him to be in agreement with me in order for this verse to work. So I read it to my husband, we agreed that we wanted a baby, and we agreed to pray about it, separately.

From that moment on, I put my barrenness in God's hands. I no longer tried to time conception. I no longer researched the causes and cures of infertility. And I no longer tried to make sense of things. Instead, I rested in the knowledge that I would receive what I asked for in prayer. It was the most peace that I had felt in years.

Little did I know, but God's plan was already in action. Within a mere week of acknowledging that my only hope of conceiving was through Him, I held a positive pregnancy test within my hands. We were healed!

The news seemed unbelievable at first, but each bout of nausea brought the wonderful reality to light. There was a baby in my womb! We had faith that we could have a baby, we asked, and we received.

Less than nine months later, my husband and I became the proud parents of a beautiful baby girl. And to this very day, she reminds us that not only is God real, but He does miraculous things for those He loves. All we needed was a bit of faith.

If you are dealing with infertility, pray to the Lord for healing. With God, all things are possible. There are many scriptural verses that support the power of faith and healing, and you can directly apply them to your situation. The Lord knows your heart.

Psalm 113:9 He settles the barren woman in her home as a happy mother of children.

Matthew 7:7-8 Ask and it will be given to you; seek and you will find; knock and the door will be opened to you. For everyone who asks receives; he who seeks finds; and to him who knocks, the door will be opened.

Matthew 17:20-21 . . . I tell you the truth, if you have faith as small as a mustard seed, you can say to this mountain, "Move from here to there," and it will move. Nothing will be impossible for you.

Matthew 21:21-22 Jesus replied, "I tell you the truth, if you have faith and do not doubt, not only can you do what was done to the fig tree, but also you can say to this mountain, 'Go, throw yourself into the sea,' and it will be done. If you believe, you will receive whatever you ask for in prayer."

Mark 9:23 . . . Everything is possible for him who believes.

James 1:6 But when he asks, he must believe and not doubt, because he who doubts is like a wave of the sea, blown and tossed by the wind.

James 5:15 And the prayer offered in faith will make the sick person well; the Lord will raise him up. If he has sinned, he will be forgiven.

Barrenness is not an obstacle for the Lord. Instead, it is a tool of the devil. The Bible gives many examples of barren, faith-filled women who conceive. The Lord has included these women in His Book as a testimony of His compassion and power.

Sarah

Genesis 11:30 Now Sarai was barren; she had no children.

Genesis 21:1-2 Now the Lord was gracious to Sarah as he had said, and the Lord did for Sarah what he had promised. Sarah became pregnant and bore a son to Abraham in his old age, at the very time God had promised him.

Rebekah

Genesis 25:21 Isaac prayed to the Lord on behalf of his wife, because she was barren. The Lord answered his prayer, and his wife Rebekah became pregnant.

Leah

Genesis 29:31 When the Lord saw that Leah was not loved, he opened her womb, but Rachel was barren.

Rachel

Genesis 30:22-23 Then God remembered Rachel; he listened to her and opened her womb. She became pregnant and gave birth to a son and said, "God has taken away my disgrace."

Manoah's Wife

Judges 13:3 The angel of the Lord appeared to her and said, "You are sterile and childless, but you are going to conceive and have a son."

Hannah

1 Samuel 1:27 I prayed for this child, and the Lord has granted me what I asked of him.

Elizabeth

Luke 1:7 But they had no children, because Elizabeth was barren; and they were both well along in years.

Luke 1:24 After this his wife Elizabeth became pregnant and for five months remained in seclusion.

God is the one who created woman and gave her the ability to bear children. Therefore, it is only natural for you to yearn for a baby because He has implanted that desire within you. It is in His Will for women to bear children. And in His eyes, it is a blessing to have many children.

Genesis 1:28 God blessed them and said to them, "Be fruitful and increase in number; fill the earth and subdue it . . . "

Exodus 23:25-26 Worship the Lord your God, and his blessing will be on your food and water. I will take away sickness from among you, and none will miscarry or be barren in your land. I will give you a full life span.

Deuteronomy 7:13-14 He will love you and bless you and increase your numbers. He will bless the fruit of your womb . . . You will be blessed more than any other people; none of your men or women will be childless, nor any of your livestock without young.

Psalm 127:3-5 Sons are a heritage from the Lord, children a reward from him. Like arrows in the hands of a warrior are sons born in one's youth. Blessed is the man whose quiver is full of them . . .

Psalm 128:3 Your wife will be like a fruitful vine within your house; your sons will be like olive shoots around your table.

So have faith and trust in the Lord. In His time, you will be the mother of many. I know that in the face of infertility it is difficult to remain hopeful, but give your fears to God and He will comfort you. Not to sound gimmicky, but if it can happen for me, it can surely happen for you. Our merciful Creator does not show favoritism.

Miscarriage

Miscarriage, without a doubt, is an awful subject for all expecting women. It is a fear that we all have and are afraid to think about. Yet considering that it occurs in approximately one out of every three pregnancies, it needs to be discussed.

Most miscarriages occur within the first trimester, usually before the baby has reached twelve weeks gestation. It often takes place before the expecting mother even knows of her pregnancy. But for those who are aware of the life inside, no matter how unformed it may be, the loss is heartbreaking.

The most common cause of an early miscarriage is said to be due to chromosomal abnormalities. There isn't anything that can be done about it, medically speaking. It is simply the body's way of stopping a defective process. It is definitely not the woman's fault.

If you are experiencing the loss of an unborn child, the most important thing to do is to take care of yourself. Eat well, drink plenty of fluids, and rest. It is crucial to relax and stay off of your feet so that you don't cause yourself to hemorrhage. Moreover, if your miscarriage is simply a threatened miscarriage, these actions will help save your baby.

Like many women, you may feel the need to see your midwife or doctor during this frightening time. An ultrasound can indicate whether the baby has passed or not. You can also be examined to verify that your body is doing what it is supposed to do. Be forewarned, however, that a doctor is likely to request an internal exam that *may* harm your unborn baby if your miscarriage is only threatened, not inevitable.

Other women, like myself, prefer staying at home. As long as you are taking care of yourself and the bleeding is under control, there is no need to be examined. What is necessary is to be aware of the process and what should and shouldn't be happening.

Depending on the woman and how far along she is, a miscarriage can manifest itself in different ways. It most commonly begins with cramping, bleeding, or both. Cramping alone does not indicate a definite miscarriage, nor does bleeding. Yet the two of them together *usually* signal the onset of the unthinkable.

The cramping may feel like regular menstrual-type pains, or more severe as in labor itself. The purpose is to clean the baby and the placenta out of the uterus. Although uncomfortable, it is a natural process that must take place. Tampons should never be used because it is vital that all of the remains be passed.

Some miscarriages begin with rupture of the membranes. This is when the bag of waters breaks. It is a clear fluid, usually, and has a distinct odor. A first-time-mother may mistake it for urine. However, if the gush of fluid is followed by cramping and bleeding, a miscarriage has occurred.

The blood flow during a miscarriage can vary, but is often like a heavy period. No more than two cups worth should be lost, otherwise the mother may become anemic. If she pays attention to what passes, the mother may find the baby or the placenta.

In early pregnancy, the baby won't look much like a baby. Instead, it may look like a blood clot, or a grayish or pinkish mass. Sometimes these remains are re-absorbed by the body. However, if any remnants are found, the mother may want to save and bury them.

Sadly, after two successful pregnancies, I experienced my first miscarriage. Here's a glimpse into one of the most horrifying moments of my life.

Everywhere I turned I was met with sympathetic smiles and gentle words. Everyone knew that my mother had recently passed. A few even came to her funeral. Everyone also knew about my new pregnancy, and I could see their minds shift from one life event to another. Their warm smiles gradually turned into all-out grins, for a congratulation was in order. And I couldn't agree more. The pregnancy was a blessing–a blessing that could not have come at a better time.

As I tucked myself behind a decorated table, balloons and streamers strewn about, I suddenly felt a gush of fluid. I assumed that it was excess discharge, and feared that it was blood. But one thing apparent was that it soaked through my clothing.

Moments later, after mustering enough courage, I slipped into the bathroom. In the absence of blood, I briefly exhaled a heavy sigh of relief. Yet something still didn't seem right. It was the distinct and unmistakable odor that filled the air. It was a scent that brought me two years back to my home-birth. It was the odor of amniotic fluid–a detrimental sign to my thirty-two-week premature baby. Gripped by fear and panic, I realized that my waters had broken. I was losing my baby.

It took all of my strength to not break down and cry. It took even more strength to open the bathroom door and step back into the lively birthday party. I was met with more congratulations, questions of how far along I was, and a dear sister-in-law who had already bought me a pair of maternity pants. It was almost more than I could bear.

There were no goodbyes that night. I just could not speak another word. I told my husband what was happening, and slipped out the door, unnoticed. My mind was whirling with terror and dread. I couldn't believe what was happening.

The following morning I began bleeding. It was light at first, but became heavier by the next day. I spent a good part of the night trying to breathe through the ongoing contractions. It reminded me of labor, but worse, because it was the delivery of a baby who had passed.

The next few days were agonizing. I worried. I waited. I hoped and prayed that the bleeding would stop. But it didn't. Each bloodied menstrual pad brought me one step closer to the reality that I so earnestly hid from. I was losing my baby.

Toward the end of that harrowing week, I noticed something on my menstrual pad. It was the placenta. About the size of my thumb nail, it was flat, oval, and a pinkish color. Dangling from it was a portion of the umbilical cord, but my baby was gone.

That very moment symbolized the end of my pregnancy. There was no more waiting. No more wondering. No more hoping. As unfair as it seemed, reality had spoken. The journey was over, and that placenta was the closest I was going to get to my baby. I admired it, and knew that it would be a moment I'd remember forever.

During my miscarriage, I sorely grieved for my baby. It occurred on the heels of my mother's death and seemed almost more than I could bear. But I remained in faith and relied on the Lord to pull me through. Most of all, I had faith in a verse that came from the mouth of Jesus.

Matthew 5:4 Blessed are those who mourn, for they will be comforted.

The Lord did comfort me. It was in Him alone that I found comfort, and I am positive that He made things easier. I also knew that one day I would get to meet my baby in Heaven. If not one hair falls off of my head that the Lord doesn't know about, then how much more important my unborn child must be to Him.

Having a miscarriage by no means indicates that you cannot carry a child. It is not your fault, and it does not make it more likely to happen again. Medically speaking, a miscarriage isn't considered abnormal until it occurs three times. At this point, a doctor may choose to explore the cause. Just remember that everything is in the Lord's control and to desire that the Lord's Will be done.

Exodus 23:25-26 Worship the Lord your God, and his blessing will be on your food and water. I will take away sickness from among you, and none will miscarry or be barren in your land. I will give you a full life span.

This verse deserves a lot of thought from those of us who have miscarried. As believers, we all worship the Lord. Even so, many of us still suffer the loss of an unborn child. It is tragic, really. But preventing this loss involves more than mere worship. It is a matter of faith. It is about believing and not doubting. It is also about choosing to stand on God's Word.

During the onset of a miscarriage, it is difficult to remain calm and faithful. Instead, you are engulfed by a raging storm of emotions. You feel fear, panic, sorrow, dread, and even helplessness. As soon as you allow these emotions to take over, they replace your faith. **In any given situation you have two choices: You can have either faith or fear. One replaces the other, and there is no room for both.** But to save your baby, you must have faith.

Matthew 14:29-31 . . . Then Peter got down out of the boat, walked on the water and came toward Jesus. But when he saw the wind, he was afraid and, beginning to sink, cried out, "Lord, save me!" Immediately Jesus reached out his hand and caught him. "You of little faith," he said, "why did you doubt?"

By faith, Peter walked on water. But with fear and doubt, he sank. The same is possible for you. You can have either faith or fear. Faith will save your baby. Fear will allow the destroyer to succeed. Faith motivates God. Fear motivates the devil. It is your choice.

James 4:7-8 Submit yourselves, then, to God. Resist the devil and he will flee from you. Come near to God and he will come near to you . . .

Scripture tells us that if we resist the devil, he will flee from us. By our resistance, he has no other choice but to flee! Consequently, if he flees, he cannot harm our unborn children. So when under attack, resist the devil and command that he leaves you alone. At the same time, draw near to God. Tell God that you will not accept anything that is not His blessing. He will comfort and protect you.

Romans 10:9-10 That if you confess with your mouth, "Jesus is Lord," and believe in your heart that God raised him from the dead, you will be saved. For it is with your heart that you believe and are justified, and it is with your mouth that you confess and are saved.

Romans 10:17 Consequently, faith comes from hearing the message, and the message is heard through the word of Christ.

A vital part of resisting the devil is to confess what you believe. To do this, you must speak aloud. You must verbally command the devil to leave you alone. You must verbally command your body to function properly and to not cast its young before its time. Confession is an affirmative way of speaking what you believe in your heart. It is also a way of building faith, because faith comes by hearing.

So during the onset of a miscarriage, or a trial of any kind, confess what you believe. Confirm to yourself where you stand. Confirm to the devil where you stand. Confirm to the Lord where you stand. Be strong, and above all, remain in faith. A miscarriage is not the Will of God. Stand on this knowledge and protect the fruit of your womb.

I offer a prayer to those of you who have experienced the loss of an unborn child. It doesn't have to happen again. It didn't have to happen to begin with. But now that we know God's stance on the subject, we can firmly and faithfully stand on His Word. God's Word says that we do not have to miscarry. If God says it, then it must be so.

Dear Heavenly Father,

Your Word says that if we worship You, we will not miscarry. It also says that if we resist the devil, he will flee from us. We believe in Your Word, Lord. We also have faith and we do not doubt. May those of us who worship You, never experience the loss of another child. Amen.

Sometimes it is very difficult to greave for a baby that you have never actually seen. It is also upsetting when the people around you push it aside as though it wasn't really a baby. It was a baby.

Talking to God is always the best way to express your feelings, especially when those close to you are not lending a listening ear. You can also find your own personal way to mourn. Different people handle things in different ways.

As for me, I spent a great deal of time in prayer. I also continued to write in a baby journal that I began shortly after discovering that I was pregnant. It allowed me to tell my baby how much I did love him or her, and it gave me something to hold on to.

My Baby Journal

January 16ᵗʰ, 2005
Week #5

Dear Baby,

Your Daddy and I were going to begin dieting this week. Since my cycle was late, which occurs often because your sister is still nursing, I took a pregnancy test. Yet to my disappointment, it appeared negative.

Although I didn't feel pregnant, something inside of me wanted that test to be positive. Maybe I am destined to be a mother of many. Maybe it is the remnant of struggling with years of infertility. Either way, I deeply wished to see two lines appear. They didn't, my hope faded, and my heart was broken.

Moments later, I took a closer look with the hope of seeing something else, and there it was! Right next to the dark control line stood a fainter one. I wasn't sure if I was really seeing it, or if it was wishful thinking. It was so faint that, at certain angles, I couldn't see it at all. But I grasped the test with both hands and stared at this barely-visible line. Excitement bubbled throughout my veins.

I called your Daddy into the bathroom and showed him the test. I was already grinning from ear to ear, and yes, he could see it too! We're having another baby! But just to be sure, I took another test later that evening. It was a definite positive. We are definitely having another baby! What wonderful news!

January 23rd, 2005
Week #6

Dear Baby,

On Tuesday, January 18th, your "Titi" passed away (my mother). It was sudden and she never had a chance to know of your existence. I am so sorry that you will never get to meet her. I am engulfed by immeasurable sorrow, but the simple thought of you growing within me brings peace. Although the life of my dear mother has vanished, another life is blooming inside of me. I am so thankful for you, dear baby of mine.

January 31st, 2005
Week #8

Dear Baby,

On Friday evening, my waters broke. It was such a horrible experience and I was terrified of losing you. Although I have only known of your existence for a couple of weeks, I love you so much. The thought of losing you and not getting to know you brings me great sorrow—more sorrow than words can express.

Saturday morning, I began bleeding. On Sunday, before daybreak, the bleeding became heavier and was accompanied by severe cramping. It was painful like labor, only worse because it was the delivery of a baby lost.

I have spent the past couple of days mourning your loss. The grief is almost unbearable. A part of my mind still deeply wishes that you have survived this horrific event. However, I don't want to have false hope. I want to be realistic. Even though it does appear that I have miscarried and that you are no longer in my aching womb, I can't help but to hold on to the hope that you are still here with me.

Dearest baby, if you have survived it is only by a miracle of the Lord. I long to see you, to hold you, to comfort you, and to just know you. You have two wonderful sisters here who are looking forward to meeting you. You also have a wonderful Daddy who has never stopped holding faith that you are still alive. I hope and pray that he is right. I love you, baby of mine, more than words can express.

February 1ˢᵗ, 2005
Week #8

Dear Baby,

As of now, I still don't know if you are here with me. What I do know is that I think of you at every waking moment and in my dreams. I love you as much as a mother could love a child. My arms ache to hold you. I just don't want to imagine life without you.

Everything that has occurred goes flashing through my mind. I grasp at any indication that you are still here—nausea, movement, anything. I can hardly eat. I can hardly sleep.

The second that I awake in the morning I think of you. My stomach knots and I am swept up into a whirlwind of sorrow. All I want is for you to live. You deserve to live. You are an innocent, unborn child. Baby, I love you so much. You will always be a part of me.

February 2ⁿᵈ, 2005
Week #8

Dear Baby,

I passed your placenta and umbilical cord today. It was small, like the size of my thumb. You were no where to be found. It was so sad to know that, at one point in time, this was your lifeline. What happened? What went wrong?

By the size of things, I can only imagine how tiny you must have been–maybe the size of my pinky nail. But none of that matters. I just can't believe that you are gone. No matter how unformed you may have been you were still my sweet baby. I love you just as much as I love your sisters. I have saved your placenta just as I have saved theirs. This spring, I will plant it in the back yard with a beautiful tree over the top–a weeping cherry. It will always remind me of your precious life.

Dearest Baby, this feels like the end. But I don't want this to be the end. I am not ready to lose hope and I am not ready to lose you. I long for the nausea to return. I want to see my feet swell and my belly grow big. I want you to know me, to know that I am your Mama, and to know that I love you.

I guess that there is no chance that you are still living within me–not unless you were a twin and your sibling has died. My mind can only imagine the possibilities, but the reality of it doesn't seem so promising. I love you.

February 2ⁿᵈ, 2005
Week #8

Dear Baby,

Sadly, I think the time has come to say goodbye. Up until now, I have continued to take my prenatal vitamins, monitor my food and activity, and record the information daily. Now that the placenta has been delivered, I think that it is safe to assume that you are gone.

I'm not sure why the Lord gave you to me for such a short time, but I am glad that He did. Maybe it was to ease the pain of my mother's death. Maybe not. But one thing that is for sure is that I love you. You are my baby and I am your Mama. A part of you is always within me.

On the outside I may appear as a mother of two, but in my heart I am the mother of three. I almost feel as though I should name you, but I don't even know if you were a girl or boy. I love you so much, sweet baby of mine. I can't say that enough. This is just so sad.

One moment I was so full of life. My dreams were filled with thoughts of you. Your Daddy's hand would gently lie on my belly. He was so proud of you already.

The next moment I was left with sadness and emptiness. Each time blood flowed from my body I was made dreadfully aware of your fate. It was like watching you die. I've spent a week watching you die.

I cried for you, but you probably didn't hear me. I mourned for you. You may have already been gone. I went from having so much to having so little.

I think of the life that you will never have. You will never be held in your Mama's arms. You will never feel the comfort of my breasts. You will never get to play with your sisters who are still anticipating your arrival. You will never get to feel the love we share in this family. It kills me to think that your little ears will never hear "I love you." But you are loved. Please know that you are loved.

I may never know the day your little heart stopped beating. I may never know what went wrong. But what I do know is that this is good-bye. It isn't a forever good-bye, but a good-bye for now. It is a good-bye until we meet again in Heaven.

It is not an overstatement to say that a parent will never *get over* the loss of a child. You don't. And it is unrealistic and insensitive of others to expect that of you. But what is so wonderful about knowing the Lord is that He can ease the pain. It doesn't hurt forever, and it isn't an end for your baby. It is only the beginning of his or her eternal life. One day, when you return to your Father in Heaven, you will get to hold that little blessing that once occupied your womb. There, the two of you will never again be separated. That is the beauty of salvation.

Chapter Two

A s a married woman of childbearing years, it is important to remember that an unexpected pregnancy could occur during any given month. With that in mind, you should generally take care of yourself as though you were already pregnant. Avoid excessive alcohol use, drugs, smoking, heavy lifting, and anything else that could negatively affect your unborn baby.

If you have decided to actively try to conceive, start by preparing your body for the journey ahead. Try to make healthier food choices and begin taking a prenatal vitamin. Also remember to avoid anything that could harm your body or your baby.

To Plan or Not To Plan?

This is a common question among many faith-filled couples who desire to do God's Will in every area of their lives, including conception. There are two main ways that natural, faith-filled parents handle the decision of when to conceive. They are known as *Quiver Full* and *Natural Family Planning*. Unlike modern birth control, both methods are completely safe.

The first method, Quiver Full, is based on the simple principle of allowing God's Will to be done. You do not try to avoid conception, nor use any form of contraception. Instead, you let nature take its course. Each month is an opportunity for pregnancy, and you accept what the Lord does or does not give you.

I can imagine how leery many of you may be of this, as I once was. You envision yourself eternally pregnant–delivering one child after another. But keep in mind that the Lord has designed your body to allow a healthy break between children. If you nurse your baby exclusively, it is highly unlikely for your menstrual cycle to return for at least six months, thus dramatically reducing the possibility of pregnancy. Also remember that the Lord knows your heart.

To me, the Quiver Full method is truly a God-honoring way of having children. Who are we to decide that we want to cut-off our seed? And how upsetting it must be to God when He chooses to bless our wombs and we naively reject our own offspring.

The second method, Natural Family Planning, involves learning your body's reproductive cycle, specifically ovulation, so that you can plan accordingly. Many believers feel that this is the responsible way to have babies. It doesn't involve any contraceptives and is merely a matter of timing. If you want to conceive, you *baby dance* (make love) within the ovulation period. If you want to avoid conception, you avoid *baby dancing* around the ovulation period. It is fairly simple, as long as you are able to interpret your own menstrual cycles.

The average menstrual cycle is approximately twenty-eight days long, with ovulation occurring around the fourteenth day. To detect ovulation, most women use a combination of methods, including precise record keeping of previous cycles, tracking basal body temperature, observing changes in cervical mucus, as well as using ovulation test strips.

Basal body temperature is a term referring to a woman's temperature first thing in the morning–*prior* to *any* activity. Before ovulation, this temperature will be about one degree Fahrenheit lower than after ovulation. Precise tracking of this temperature over a period of time will give a woman insight as to how *her* menstrual cycle operates.

For women who are more in-tune with their bodies, observing changes in cervical mucus often proves to be a very accurate indication that ovulation is near. Prior to ovulation, a noticeable change occurs in a woman's cervical mucus, for it becomes thick and stretchy–quite comparable to egg-white. Conception is likely to occur around this time.

And finally, there are ovulation test strips. These test strips work similarly to pregnancy test strips, only they detect the luteinizing hormone (LH) in urine instead of human chorionic gonadotropin (HCG). LH is always present in urine, but briefly and dramatically rises prior to ovulation. This is known as the LH surge, and is a very accurate indication of ovulation.

For those of you who currently use modern birth control, be forewarned that you may be inadvertently aborting your own babies. Regardless of what you may have been told, most forms of the Pill and the intrauterine device (IUD), among others, *do not* prevent pregnancy. Instead, they *abort* pregnancy *after* it has already occurred.

It is probable that modern birth control destroys more unborn babies each year than surgical abortions. In light of this, each woman must reconsider the consequences of her actions. There are safer ways to prevent pregnancy, and it is vital to choose a method that does not recklessly endanger the lives of unborn children.

Are You Pregnant?

As my past miscarriage has taught me, early pregnancy does *feel* a certain way. It is too subtle of a sensation to put into words, but it is just as real as the pregnancy itself. Matter of fact, the sudden absence of this *feeling*, such as in a miscarriage, is more noticeable. You notice that you don't *feel* pregnant anymore, even if you didn't *feel* pregnant to begin with.

Once conception occurs, some women "just know" that they are pregnant. They may recognize little signs from their past pregnancies, or have a subconscious awareness of symptoms that are not yet apparent. Either way, they are usually correct in their intuitive assumptions.

On the other hand, some women experience a slight inkling that something is going on, or that something has changed, yet remain unsure until a definite sign appears. They may briefly ponder the idea of being pregnant, but brush it off as wishful thinking.

And finally, there are women who have absolutely no idea that they may be pregnant until they have missed a period. Then, and only then, do they feel prompted to take a pregnancy test.

The symptoms of early pregnancy are often difficult to detect, and most women will simply feel *different*. They *may* feel tired, nauseated, or emotional. They *may* notice the enlargement of their breasts or a feeling of fullness in their abdomens. Or, they *may* notice nothing at all. A positive pregnancy test is the only sure way to know.

With my first pregnancy, I remember feeling so exhausted one day that I couldn't even finish showering standing up. Instead, I sat on the floor to shampoo and condition my hair.

Immediately afterwards, I wrapped myself in a bath towel, laid on my bed, and awoke about four hours later. This bout of fatigue was unexplainable, and in hindsight, it was my first "official" pregnancy symptom.

With my second pregnancy, I just felt pregnant. Even though two pregnancy tests showed that I wasn't, I still insisted that I was. I wasn't tired at all, but I did begin experiencing morning sickness. About a week later, I finally tested positive.

With my third (successful) pregnancy, as you will read in my baby journal, I just awoke one morning with the strange desire to take a pregnancy test. I did, and the faintest line appeared.

In the end, there is no surefire way to know if you are pregnant except for a positive pregnancy test. However, if you intuitively feel that you are pregnant, then you most likely are.

The most productive time to take a urine pregnancy test is first thing in the morning. This is due to the concentrated levels of HCG that would be present. Depending on how far long you are, a positive result may appear immediately.

Although most pregnancy test manufacturers recommend that the results should be acquired within a certain time period to ensure accuracy, my experience has been different. Sometimes a test that appears negative within the allotted time may become positive later. Even the faintest line indicates a positive result. If this occurs, retest in a day or so to confirm the results.

If the test still appears negative an hour or so later, but you feel pregnant, simply retest in a day or so. It is more cost-efficient to purchase HCG pregnancy test strips online or at a dollar store if you plan to test often.

For those of you who have experienced a recent miscarriage, it is likely that pregnancy hormones are still circulating throughout your body. These hormones could trigger a positive result even a month or so later, all dependent on how far along you were. Please keep this in mind to save yourself from further disappointment.

When Are You Due?

Congratulations! You have a baby on the way and you care enough about this unborn child to want to do things naturally. This is the most positive step that you can take for both you and your child. So where do you begin?

The most obvious place is to calculate your estimated date of delivery (EDD). To do this, we use a method called *Naegele's Rule.* You count back three months from the first day of your last menstrual period and add one week. However, keep in mind that this date is only an estimate. Your baby can safely be born as early as thirty-seven weeks gestation. Although forty-two weeks gestation is the cut-off point, many women, myself included, exceed that without complication.

Where to Deliver?

When it comes to pregnancy, you must first remember that God is in control. He designed your body specifically for this purpose. There is no need to feel alarmed or to rush to the nearest doctor. You are in good hands and your baby is as safe as it could possibly be.

The first step is to decide where you want to deliver. To determine this, you should ask the Lord for guidance and sincerely try to understand His view on childbirth. How does He, the Creator, want it to be handled? And is it okay for women to prostitute their bodies to men who carry a man-made title such as *doctor* or *obstetrician*?

Childbirth *is* meant to be a personal and profound part of a woman's life, only to be shared by her most intimate friends and family members. If God had intended it to be any other way, babies would not be born from the most private part of a woman's body.

Childbirth *is not* a medical emergency, an illness, nor a spectator sport with free admission to the medical community. Yet the field of modern medicine has turned it into these things and more.

Matthew 9:12 On hearing this, Jesus said, "It is not the healthy who need a doctor, but the sick."

Although Jesus used this phrase to emphasize that it is the sinner He is calling, not the righteous, it still proves an important point. In His time, it was common knowledge that doctors were for the sick. With that said, pregnancy is not an illness and therefore does not require the services of a doctor.

In this country, however, the most common place to deliver a baby is in a hospital with a doctor. Consequently, it is also the most common place to end up with complications that could have been prevented by not intervening. Yet with this being a book for natural, faith-filled parents, it is safe to assume that you will want to avoid what modern medicine has to offer unless absolutely necessary.

Exodus 1:15-17 The king of Egypt said to the Hebrew midwives, whose names were Shiphrah and Puah, "When you help the Hebrew women in childbirth and observe them on the delivery stool, if it is a boy, kill him; but if it is a girl, let her live." The midwives, however, feared God and did not do what the king of Egypt had told them to do; they let the boys live.

In biblical times, midwives were the ones who delivered babies. The word *midwife* means *with wife,* or in other words, *with woman.* Midwives weren't men, they were women. God chose women to deliver the babies of other women, and no one else would be better suited. So where did men come into the picture?

When medicine became the money-driven profession that it is today, *only* men were allowed to educate themselves and earn the required credentials. Out of greed, these men decided to make childbirth into a medical event, thus barring midwives from legally delivering babies. This monopoly left birthing women with one choice: To deliver their babies in a hospital with a doctor. What a deceitful marketing strategy on the part of the medical profession!

Fortunately, midwifery has stood the test of time. It was the Lord's original intent to have women helping women through childbirth, and it is making a comeback. But are the midwives of today the same as the midwives of yesterday? The answer is yes and no.

Traditional midwives train by apprenticeship. They have a passion for birth and a sincere trust in the female body. They also deeply care for their clients and put them and their unborn children above all else.

Certified midwives are another story. Although there are many wonderful certified midwives, there are equally as many who are more medically inclined. These midwives are bridging the needed gap between natural and unnatural birth. And, the results are alarming. They may eventually mesh with modern medicine and inadvertently eradicate midwifery. This is especially true with the emergence of male-midwives.

What concerns me with midwifery in general is that it often has new-age tendencies. Many midwives are God-fearing, and many are not. Those who are not believers in God frequently dabble in unnatural practices. It is here where the natural and unnatural clash. These pagan midwives support yoga, meditation, and a host of other non-biblical ways.

In choosing a midwife, whether traditional or certified, it is up to your discretion to locate a God-fearing one. It is, however, well-worth the effort. Many midwives are dedicated and compassionate women with a lot to offer. The area of childbirth is indeed better because of them.

Unfortunately, midwifery care is not the norm in our society. Women have been deliberately misled into believing that a doctor-assisted hospital birth is the safest and most acceptable choice. This notion couldn't be further from the truth. Women have also been deceived into believing that it is acceptable to submit their bodies to *anyone* who carries a man-made title.

Hebrews 13:4 Marriage should be honored by all, and the marriage bed kept pure, for God will judge the adulterer and all the sexually immoral.

As the above verse plainly states, marriage should be honored by *all*. Once a couple unites, the wife belongs to her husband, and the husband to his wife. It is sexually immoral and adulterous for either partner to offer their body *outside* of the marriage. Pregnancy and childbirth are no exception.

Some may argue that a doctor isn't just any man, and that it is acceptable for a woman, married or not, to submit to his every request. Some may also argue that a doctor is not performing sexual tasks, but medical ones. Yet under whose authority is he doing these things?

The fact that a doctor holds a man-ordained certificate does not make his behavior appropriate or acceptable. It is wrong for a woman to allow a man, besides her husband, to fondle with her body in any way, and especially in a sexually-oriented manner. For this very reason, God appointed midwives to care for women during pregnancy and childbirth.

Male doctors are unacceptable for childbirth simply due to

their gender, while female doctors pose other problems. Just like their male counterparts, their training causes them to view everything with medically-shaded glasses. They consider childbirth a dangerous medical event and will treat it as such. Their unnecessary interventions can and will endanger the life of you and your baby. It is *not* okay to needlessly put yourself or your baby in harm's way.

So with that said, midwives are clearly a God-honoring way of handling childbirth. They allow nature to take its course, thus letting God's Will be done. But besides midwives, are there other ways? And how does God feel about a couple delivering their own children, as many faith-filled believers now do?

Luke 2:5-7 He went there to register with Mary, who was pledged to be married to him and was expecting a child. While they were there, the time came for the baby to be born, and she gave birth to her firstborn, a son. She wrapped him in cloths and placed him in a manger, because there was no room for them in the inn.

Jesus is the Son of God. He lived on this earth as one of us, and we are to live by His example. As we read the above verse, Jesus was obviously not delivered by a doctor. It appears that a midwife wasn't present either. Instead, His birth was God-assisted. This was the way that our Lord chose for His one and only Son to be born. That says a lot in itself.

In-Hospital Birthing Centers

For those of you who feel that you require a hospital birth, it is good to know that many now have built-in birthing centers with midwives. Here, you will increase the likelihood of experiencing a safe and natural birth, opposed to delivering in a traditional maternity ward. And it is definitely a safer option, but one that still concerns me.

Considering that you are still within a hospital, you would be more likely to fall victim to unnecessary intervention. In addition to that, the birthing center would not be independent and therefore still subject to hospital regulations. Although you *may* achieve a natural birth, you will be coerced into accepting routine procedures such as vaccinations, the vitamin K injection, the eye ointment, and multiple tests. Be sure to weight the positive and negative aspects carefully.

Freestanding Birthing Centers

A safer alternative is to deliver in a freestanding birthing center. Here, you will have regular prenatal appointments with one of the employed midwives. They usually rotate your visits so that you can get to know each one in preparation for the birth.

The midwives in a freestanding birthing center tend to be very compassionate women with a sincere interest in you and your pregnancy. They are well-trained with extensive knowledge of the female body and the birth process. More than anything, they want to help you have a safe and satisfying birth experience. And unlike doctors, midwives have been delivering babies since biblical times.

The atmosphere in a freestanding birthing center is often very laid back and pleasant. You will have access to many routine tests and procedures with the option to refuse. You will also be close to a hospital in the event of an emergency. For those of you who aren't comfortable with overseeing your own pregnancy, midwives are a wonderful choice with promising results.

Home-Birth Midwives

A similar option is a home-birth midwife. She performs all of your routine prenatal care and attends the delivery. The difference is that you are able to deliver in the comfort and privacy of your own home.

Most home-birth midwives are very relaxed and have the utmost confidence in the female body. They are also more likely to be open to the complete avoidance of routine procedures. With that in mind, they are especially valuable to women who have suffered any form of sexual abuse. Home-birth midwives are often willing to perform all of your prenatal care without overstepping your boundaries. Unfortunately, depending on where you live, their practice may be illegal. But this does not mean that they do not exist.

Unassisted Home-Births

A final option is to deliver your baby at home, unassisted. But as believers, we aren't really unassisted, but God-assisted. And this is, after all, the way He chose for His one and only Son to be born.

The decision to have an unassisted home-birth isn't one to take lightly. You must first examine your motives and determine what you want out of the experience. Like myself, maybe you have had a traumatic birth and long for healing. Maybe this is your first pregnancy and you are learning from the mistakes of the women before you. Or maybe your first birth wasn't horrifying, but it wasn't satisfying either. The possibilities are endless, but regardless of your reason, it is valid.

An unassisted home-birth isn't for everyone. If you want someone else to manage your pregnancy, labor, and delivery, it isn't for you. You belong in a hospital or birthing center. If you want pain medication, the reassurance of medical professionals, and a host of tests and internal exams, again, delivering at home isn't the way to go.

On the other hand, if you are an independent woman with faith in the Lord and confidence in your body, delivering at home, unassisted, may be for you. If you deeply care about your baby, and your baby's health is more important than your comfort, an unassisted home-birth is ideal.

The reasons to have this type of birth go beyond avoiding toxins and interventions. It is about taking responsibility for you and the life inside of you. It is also about respecting your baby and yourself and not offering either of you as a playing field for medical technology. Most important, it is an act of faith.

Delivering a baby at home, unassisted, is legal in most

states. The father is usually labeled as the *baby catcher*, unless the mother attempts it alone. The legal requirements do vary, so be sure of your state's laws.

Before making the important and possibly life-altering decision of where to deliver, carefully research your options and ask the Lord to show you the way. This isn't the time to be passive or compliant with the wishes of other's. This also is not the time to just go with the flow. It is crucial that you make the best choice for you and your unborn baby. Both of your lives depend on it.

Prenatal Care

If you have chosen to do prenatal care through a midwife, she will help guide you in the right direction. However, be sure to research everything for yourself. The decisions that you will need to make are far too important to rely on someone else's word or opinion.

For those of you who have chosen to do an unassisted home-birth, or are undecided, now is the time to begin your own prenatal care. I've listed a few staples that I feel are of importance, but by no means is this an all-inclusive guide. My purpose is to pass down the simple knowledge I've gained through research and experience, just as I would to my own daughters. However, it is up to you to educate yourself.

I've included a sample prenatal checklist at the end of this chapter to help assist you in your record keeping. You may copy it if you wish, or create a similar chart on your personal computer.

Weight

The first step is to begin monitoring and charting your weight on a weekly basis. The general guideline is to gain between twenty and forty pounds within the duration of your pregnancy. Some midwives estimate that a woman should gain about one pound per week. Either way, as long as you are gradually gaining, there is no need for concern.

During early pregnancy, a woman's weight will often remain steady due to frequent bouts of nausea. Other women may gain very slowly in the beginning, and more rapidly later on. Both scenarios are normal, and not a cause for concern. As long as the woman is properly nourished, the baby is getting all that he or she needs.

Sudden and excessive weight gain may indicate an underlying problem, such as preeclampsia. If this occurs, a midwife should be contacted for further diagnosis.

Blood Pressure

Along with your weight, you should also monitor and chart your blood pressure. This is an excellent indicator that everything is progressing smoothly. You can purchase your own device or use the one at your local drug store. However, measure in the same way each time so that your results are consistent.

When taking your blood pressure, there are two measurements. The systolic reading, which is the higher number, indicates the pressure in your arteries when your heart is pumping. The diastolic reading, which is the lower number, indicates the pressure in your heart at rest.

During pregnancy, normal blood pressure levels can range from 90/50 to 140/90. However, if you notice your blood pressure on the rise, or have reached 130/80, you should take preventative measures to lower it.

Two simple ways to lower blood pressure are to do moderate exercise and reduce stress. More significantly, you should reevaluate your diet. A poor diet, based on animal products and processed foods, is probably the culprit.

Diet

When it comes to pregnancy, you cannot underestimate the

importance of what you eat. Diet is the foundation of optimal health, and specific measures must be taken to ensure that your's is complete.

Unfortunately, this can prove to be very stressful and confusing, even for the most educated of parents. Diet is a much-talked-about subject, and the conflicting information is abounding.

However, as with all things, the truth behind this mystery lies within the Bible itself. God wants for all people to be healthy, and the blueprints for achieving this have been around from the very beginning.

Genesis 1:29-30 Then God said, "I give you every seed-bearing plant on the face of the whole earth and every tree that has fruit with seed in it. They will be yours for food. And to all the beasts of the earth and all the birds of the air and all the creatures that move on the ground–everything that has the breath of life in it–I give every green plant for food." And it was so.

God's original diet for man was a complete vegan diet. There was no hunting, killing, or eating of flesh. Instead, man lived in harmony with nature and ate the food that the Lord had provided. This lifestyle supplied *all* of man's nutritional needs, and not a single illness was recorded in the Bible at that time.

Fortunately, we, too, can achieve optimal health by returning to this diet. It is based on the simple principle that the body is a living organism that requires living food. Living food is raw food. This is the basis for not only sustaining your life, but in the creation of new life.

When it comes to selecting these living foods, remember that quality counts. Choose fruits and vegetables that are organic–free of pesticides, herbicides, mold inhibitors, and genetic modification. Also be sure to select organic, whole grains, instead of the processed, nutrient-deficient versions that are so prevalent in mainstream supermarkets.

As for animal products, such as meat, fish, dairy, and eggs, they have *no* place in the ideal human diet. These substances, in addition to sugars and processed foods, account for the majority of illnesses that plague society today, ranging from the common cold to cancer. Even organic, free-range animal products are not fit for human consumption, but may be consumed sparingly with minimal effects. Be sure to follow the Levitical food laws regarding clean and unclean creatures.

The dairy industry is responsible for promoting the fallacy that milk is essential to human health. They've launched a successful marketing ploy that targets not only pregnant and nursing women, but the general public as well. What they have failed to promote is the hard fact that *most* people are allergic to dairy. Humans are the only creatures who consume the milk of other mammals, and we are reaping the results.

Allergic reactions to dairy include ADHD, Chron's disease, depression, ear infections, eczema, hives, infertility, and PMS, just to name a *few*. Milk also has amazing weight-gaining properties intended to support the massive growth of a calf within the first year of life. Any human who gains weight at the rate of a calf will become obese.

Despite popular belief, dairy is *not* essential to human health. It is definitely not the number one source of calcium available to man, for carrots and spinach have from ten to forty times *more*! Matter of fact, most nutrients in milk are destroyed in the pasteurization process, leaving it useless. Added calcium is usually inorganic, making it unusable as well.

As a pregnant woman, it is normal to be conscious about consuming an adequate amount of nutrients for your growing baby. The surefire way to do this is to rely on our Creator and His original diet for man–one of raw fruits and vegetables. Father knows best.

In addition to these raw fruits and vegetables, water is another vital substance. The body requires water for each and every function. Because of this, you should consume the purest water available. This is made possible by the distillation process, which removes all inorganic minerals. Consume distilled water liberally.

Because the earth is no longer as nutrient-dense as it once was, supplementation is wise in order to compensate for areas your diet may be lacking. The most traditional means is in the form of a prenatal vitamin, which should be purchased at a natural food store to ensure the quality.

A better alternative is to take a barley grass supplement. Barley grass contains a broad spectrum of vitamins, minerals, and amino acids that are 100% useable by the human body, unlike the inorganic substances found in a traditional vitamin.

In addition to diet, many herbs have been proven to be very beneficial in supporting a healthy pregnancy. Among the most popular are alfalfa, comfrey, dandelion leaf, nettle leaf, red clover leaves and blossoms, and red raspberry leaf. A combination of these herbs will help to support your pregnancy and entire reproductive system in immeasurable ways. Simply mix the desired amount of each herb, such as a teaspoon, steep in boiled water for at least fifteen minutes, and drink as a tea.

In the end, a health-promoting diet is the most important measure you can take to ensure the well-being of your unborn child. Make the foundation of each meal you consume the living foods that give life, and rest in the knowledge that you are giving your baby the very best.

Rest and Exercise

Rest and exercise are also important factors. If possible, nap when you are feeling tired, especially in the early months. As for exercise, do as you see fit. It is clearly not advisable to go bungee-jumping or rock-climbing, but other activities are suitable. Walking and swimming tend to be the greatest forms of exercise. They give you a well-rounded workout without too much strain. There are also DVD's available with various pregnancy-safe routines, including aerobics. Choose one that best suits you and your level of fitness.

Mid-pregnancy is a wonderful time to begin preparing for the labor and delivery. Decide what comfort measures you plan to use, and practice them beforehand. There are also simple exercises that will aid in the actual delivery of your baby. Both labor and delivery exercises are outlined in Chapter Four.

Baby's Movements

Once you reach twenty-eight weeks gestation, you should frequently and easily feel your baby moving around. Begin recording the movements daily. You will learn what to expect from your little blessing, and this is a perfect way to check up on him or her.

If a time comes when your baby seems unusually quiet, try drinking a little juice or something sugary to promote movement. If the baby still hasn't perked up, or you notice a complete cessation of movement, immediately contact a midwife.

As your baby grows, he or she will begin crowding your belly. This lack of space will limit his or her movements. During the final trimester, do not panic at the absence of large movements. Instead, pay more attention to the frequency, opposed to the strength.

Daily Prayer

Daily prayer is essential to your overall well-being. It can ease pregnancy anxiety, prevent unforeseen complications, and heal even the worst of conditions. No prenatal care regimen would be complete without it.

Set up specific times each day to pray for your pregnancy and unborn child. Build your faith by reading the Word of God, and recite verses pertaining to pregnancy and childbirth. If you've suffered a previous miscarriage, pray for emotional healing and for the vitality of your current pregnancy. If you have other concerns, or desires, pray for those too.

In Addition . . .

Do your research! Know what to expect and pay close attention to your body and your baby. If you are unsure of anything, look into it. The Internet is a very valuable resource, and there are also many wonderful books available.

Some women choose to take their prenatal care to a higher level, and you must make your own decision. From blood work, to ultrasounds, internal exams, and a urinalysis, take it to the extent that you feel comfortable.

Other women take a more relaxed approach. Faith and daily prayer are the only necessary assets. If you put the Lord first, He will crown your efforts with success. Ultimately, He is in control.

Prenatal Checklist	Sun	Mon	Tue	Wed	Thu	Fri	Sat
Weight							
Blood Pressure							
Prenatal Vitamin							
Barley Supplement							
Regular Exercise							
Labor Prep Exercises							
Delivery Prep Exercises							
Baby's Movements							
Daily Prayer							

Chapter Three

As an expecting mother, it is important for you to know what is going on inside of your body. Some women choose to take a passive approach and allow a doctor to monitor the pregnancy and make all of the necessary decisions. This can prove to be very dangerous.

Other women–thinking women, take an active approach. They know what to expect and research all that they don't understand. They also make informed decisions about every aspect of their care.

Pregnancy: What to Expect

The average duration of a pregnancy is approximately forty weeks, or nine months. As mentioned earlier, some babies are born safely at thirty-seven weeks gestation, while others are delivered well beyond their due dates. It really depends on the woman's cycle, the date of conception, the baby's development, and other factors.

The nine months of pregnancy are split into trimesters: The first trimester (the first three months); the second trimester (the second three months); and the third trimester (the last three months).

Of all the trimesters, the first is often the most challenging for a mother-in-waiting. It is a time of worry, anticipation, and the onset of unpleasant symptoms. However, it is also a time of joy and excitement. There are people to tell, things to buy, and names to sift through.

From this point on, the way that you choose to perceive pregnancy will greatly impact the road ahead. If you view it as the blessing it really is, it will be a blessing. Likewise, if you view it as a burden, it will be a burden. It is your choice.

As the second trimester arrives, many of your early pregnancy symptoms will have ceased. The time has come to relax, browse maternity clothes, and simply enjoy being pregnant.

If you are seeing a midwife, you have probably had the pleasure of hearing your baby's heartbeat. If not, you can purchase a fetal Doppler, stethoscope, or similar instrument. Most professional-quality devices work well. However, avoid anything you may come across in a mainstream store, for they are often useless until late in the last trimester.

If you choose to invest in a heart-listening device, it may take some getting used to. Try not to be alarmed if you can't find your baby's heartbeat on the first try. It does take practice. The difficulty is determined by how far along you are, your weight, and the position of the baby and the placenta.

Using a quality Doppler, you may be able to detect your baby's heartbeat as early as nine weeks gestation, but more likely at twelve weeks or later. On average, your baby's heart will beat about 120 to180 times per minute. As the old midwife's tale goes: A slower rate is a boy and a faster rate is a girl! Keep in mind, however, that this rate will gradually decrease as your pregnancy progresses, although it should remain within the 120 to 180 beats per minute range.

Once you locate your baby's heartbeat, remember that it may sound disturbing to the untrained ear. It may seem irregular, unusually fast, or suddenly stop, which simply means that the baby has changed position and you need to readjust your device. Sometimes technology causes more worry than anything else. However, if you are truly concerned, do not hesitate to contact a professional.

Once you have reached the final phase of your pregnancy, the third trimester, you may be flooded with mixed emotions. You may feel well-prepared and eager for the baby's arrival, or just the opposite. You may feel that the time is near and you have so much left to do. Be patient. There is still time for preparation, and the baby will be here soon.

The third trimester may bring on new pregnancy discomforts. The size of your growing baby puts a lot of strain on your body, and may cause back pain, muscle cramps, tiredness, and the need to empty your bladder often. You may also begin developing colostrum, a yellowish, sticky substance that will be your baby's first food.

Another issue that you may be dealing with are Braxton-Hicks contractions. These contractions can become quite intense and cause you to wonder if you are in labor. If it is true labor, the contractions will progress, becoming stronger and longer, with shorter breaks in between.

On the other hand, if you aren't experiencing true labor, use these contractions to practice relaxation techniques. It may feel frustrating or discouraging to know that you are not actually in labor, but keep in mind that your body is warming up. It is practicing for the challenge ahead, and the more contractions you have, the better prepared you will be.

Pregnancy has its ups and downs, but it will all balance out. It is a time to learn more about yourself and your body. It is a time to make changes in your life that will be better for your child. And it is a time to watch your belly grow and enjoy how beautiful you look. Everything about pregnancy is beautiful, miraculous, and inspiring.

The following chart lists the most common pregnancy complaints, when they are most likely to occur, the cause, and ways to help. You may experience all of these symptoms at one time or another, or only a few. You may also experience less common ones that aren't listed. If something worrisome does occur, just remember that with a little research, most fears can be put to rest.

Common Pregnancy Complaints

Complaint	When It Occurs	Cause	Solution
Abdominal Muscle Separation	Mid to late pregnancy	Pressure from the uterus	It will disappear after pregnancy
Backache	Late pregnancy	Bodily changes	Pelvic Rock St. John's Wort
Breast Tenderness	Early pregnancy	Hormones Increase in size	Wear a supportive bra
Colostrum	From the fifth month on	It's your baby's first food!	Wear nursing pads if necessary
Constipation	Mid to late pregnancy	Hormones Diet	Drink more fluid Eat more fiber Psyllium Seed
Diarrhea	Throughout pregnancy	Hormones Stomach flu	Drink fluids
Gum Problems	Mid to late pregnancy	Hormones Increased volume of circulation Lack of vit. C	Gentle brushing Vitamin C

Headaches	Throughout pregnancy	Random reasons Dehydration	Chamomile Cold cloth
Heartburn	Mid to late pregnancy	Baby's growth Slower digestion	Eat smaller meals Slippery Elm* Papaya
Hemorrhoids	Mid to late pregnancy	Pressure from the uterus Increased volume of circulation	Red Clover Nettle Raw Potato*** Witch Hazel
Hip Soreness	Late pregnancy	Sleeping on your side Stretching ligaments	Change position
Indigestion	Mid to late pregnancy	Baby's growth Slower digestion	Eat smaller meals Slippery Elm* Papaya
Itchiness	Late pregnancy	Stretching skin	Moisturizer
Leg Cramps	Mid to late pregnancy	Lack of calcium due to slow absorption	Calcium Massage
Ligament Pain	Throughout pregnancy	Stretching ligaments	Avoid quick movements
Morning Sickness/ Nausea	Any time of day in early pregnancy	Hormones Empty stomach Emotions	Crackers Plain yogurt Ginger tea
Nosebleeds	Throughout pregnancy	Increased volume of circulation	Vitamin C Humidifier

Pelvic Discomfort	Mid to late pregnancy	Hormones Relaxed muscles Weight of baby	Heating pad Massage Change position
Skin Changes (Pigment)	Mid to late pregnancy	Hormones	It will disappear after pregnancy
Stretch Marks	Late pregnancy	Stretched skin to accommodate growth	Vitamin E** Vitamin C Cocoa butter
Swelling of Hands and Feet	Mid to late pregnancy	Water retention Impaired circulation Long periods of standing or sitting	Elevate feet Drink water Avoid tight clothing
Tiredness	Early or late pregnancy	Hormones	Eat well Rest
Urinary Incontinence	Late pregnancy	Weak pelvic floor Weight of baby	Kegels
Vaginal Discharge	Throughout pregnancy	Increased fluids Hormones	Cotton panties Air circulation
Varicose Veins	Mid to late pregnancy	Slow circulation Hormones	Exercise Vitamin E**
Yeast Infection	Throughout pregnancy	Increased fluids Hormones	Cotton panties Tampons soaked in acidophilus

*Slippery Elm can be purchased as lozenges at a natural food store
**Vitamin E: about 400 IU daily
***The raw potato should be peeled, grated, and placed directly on the hemorrhoids

Before reaching the thirty-seventh week of your pregnancy,

you will want to have finished making the final preparations for your labor and delivery. If you are seeing a midwife, now is an excellent time to ask anything that concerns you. You will also want to write and review your *birth plan* with her. It will help ensure that there aren't any last minute surprises.

A birth plan is basically a description of how you would like for your labor and delivery to be handled. You can make it as simple or as detailed as you wish. You should include whom you want in the room during the delivery, what you plan to do for pain management, and what will be done with baby afterwards.

Problems in Pregnancy

Most women who take a non-interventionist approach to pregnancy, labor, and delivery seldom encounter major complications along the way. The road is usually a very smooth one, with a non-eventful bump here or there. This good fortune can be contributed to the fact that most natural mothers tend to be faith-filled, health-conscious women.

However, sometimes complications do arise. It can happen to the best of us. And if you are managing your own prenatal care, it is wise to know at least a little about what could occur. In light of this, I've included a *brief* description of complications that could arise during pregnancy. By no means is this a complete guide.

Vaginal bleeding in the first trimester of pregnancy occurs in approximately one out of every four women. As alarming as this may be, only one in ten of these women will actually miscarry. This type of miscarriage is known as a *spontaneous abortion.* If the membranes rupture or the cervix dilates, then an *inevitable abortion* has occurred.

Bleeding within the first half of pregnancy–especially if accompanied by a persistent backache or cramping, is known as a *threatened abortion.* As the term suggests, an actual miscarriage is possible–or threatened, but not inevitable. The blood loss may be light to moderate and continuous for days–even weeks.

Sometimes light and continuous bleeding is caused by a *missed abortion*. This is when the baby has died but remains in the mother's body. Many women will notice a complete cessation of pregnancy-related symptoms when this has occurred.

Another cause of bleeding is an *ectopic pregnancy*. This is when the placenta implants itself outside of the uterus–most commonly in one of the fallopian tubes (a *tubal pregnancy*). Symptoms of a tubal pregnancy include pelvic pain and spotting. This is a very serious situation that requires immediate medical attention.

Placental problems are also possible culprits for bleeding during pregnancy. *Placental abruption* is when the placenta prematurely separates from the uterine wall. Symptoms may include bleeding and abdominal pain.

Other placental problems are due to the actual location or position of the placenta. *Placenta praevia* is when the placenta is implanted low in the uterus. A common symptom is bleeding without abdominal pain. There are four main types of placenta praevia: A *total praevia,* which is when the placenta completely covers the cervix; a *partial praevia,* which is when the placenta partially covers the cervix; a *marginal praevia,* which is when the edge of the placenta is at the edge of the cervix; and a *low-lying placenta*, which is when the placenta is close to the cervix, but not actually reaching it.

Some pregnancy complications do not involve bleeding or pain. *Anemia*, for example, is characterized by fatigue and pallor (an unhealthy pale appearance). A woman may become anemic when she has a shortage of red cells or hemoglobin in her blood. The most common type, *iron-deficiency anemia*, is self explanatory. Simple remedies include increasing the mother's iron intake, along with protein to help build new red blood cells. It is also wise for the mother to take Vitamin C to help in iron absorption.

Gestational diabetes is a term for decreased glucose tolerance during pregnancy. There are tests available to detect gestational diabetes, including a glucose screen or an oral glucose tolerance test. One indication that gestational diabetes may be present is a fetus who is notably large for gestational age (*macrosomia*).

Hypertension is a term for high blood pressure, characterized by readings of 140/90 or higher. Prolonged hypertension can cause major complications with the baby, so it is vital to treat it immediately. A few suggestions are for the mother to exercise, avoid stimulants, eat a healthy diet, and either eliminate stress or practice relaxation techniques.

Preeclampsia is a condition characterized by generalized edema (swelling), sudden and excessive weight gain, hypertension, and protein in the urine. It is a very serious condition and requires immediate care.

Polyhydramnios and *Hydramnios* are terms referring to excess amniotic fluid. There are many causes such as twins, diabetes, and toxemia. It can cause complications such as postpartum hemorrhage, placental abruption, or uterine dysfunction.

Oligohydramnios is just the opposite of the above terms. It refers to a small amount of amniotic fluid. It may indicate underlying problems, but can sometimes be resolved by increasing fluid intake.

Toxoplasmosis is a condition that can cause severe neurological damage to a baby if it is contracted after ten weeks gestation. To avoid contracting toxoplasmosis, the mother should avoid uncooked meat and cat feces.

And finally, *postdatism*. This is a term for a pregnancy that goes beyond forty-two weeks gestation. There is a higher risk for the baby, but as long as the mother and baby are doing well, there isn't too much need for concern.

One cannot underestimate the importance of diet–especially when it comes to pregnancy. Many complications, such as gestational diabetes, hypertension, and preeclampsia can be prevented. It is vital to feed your body what it needs–raw fruits and vegetables. It is also important to limit or avoid foods that degenerate your body–sugars, white flours, and animal products.

Spiritual Preparation

Whether you are a first-time mother or an experienced veteran, spiritual preparation is a must. And although I am a firm believer in being informed, I stand firmer in relying on faith. Information will *help* you, but faith will *save* you.

If you enter pregnancy expecting bad things, you will be plagued by bad things. It is like giving the devil a foothold. But if you enter pregnancy joyfully and full of faith, your faith will carry you through unscathed. And so each pregnancy presents itself as a perfect opportunity to build your faith.

Matthew 14:29-31 . . . Then Peter got down out of the boat, walked on the water and came toward Jesus. But when he saw the wind, he was afraid and, beginning to sink, cried out, "Lord, save me!" Immediately Jesus reached out his hand and caught him. "You of little faith," he said, "why did you doubt?"

Although I have used this verse before, it does give a clear picture of what can be done with faith. It also shows what happens when you lose faith. During pregnancy, you do not want to lose faith. It is of critical importance and will enable your body and your mind to act flawlessly.

Romans 10:17 Consequently, faith comes from hearing the message, and the message is heard through the word of Christ.

Building faith isn't a difficult task, but one that requires dedication. You must surround yourself in the Word of God at all times and let nothing lead you astray. You must read and study your

Bible. You must pray to the Lord and listen for His answer. You must remove all moral filth and clothe yourself in His Word. Replace secular music with Christian music. Memorize Scripture, especially those verses pertaining to faith and childbirth. Let God be the first thing you think of when you awake, and the last before falling asleep. Be prayerful about everything and watch your tongue. Do not unintentionally curse yourself.

Ephesians 4:22-24 You were taught, with regard to your former way of life, to put off your old self, which is being corrupted by its deceitful desires; to be made new in the attitude of your minds; and to put on the new self, created to be like God in true righteousness and holiness.

Pregnancy is an excellent time to *put on the new self.* You should rid your mind of all doubt and the worldly notions surrounding childbirth. Instead, wrap yourself in the Lord's Word and aim to do everything that pleases Him.

Proverbs 3:5-6 Trust in the Lord with all your heart and lean not on your own understanding; in all your ways acknowledge him, and he will make your paths straight.

Similarly, do not lean on your own understanding. Human understanding is unstable and easily clouded by preconceived notions and traditions. Don't fall victim to that. Instead, trust in the Lord. Put Him first in everything you do and He will make your paths straight.

Romans 10:9-10 That if you confess with your mouth, "Jesus is Lord," and believe in your heart that God raised him from the dead, you will be saved. For it is with your heart that you believe and are justified, and it is with your mouth that you confess and are saved.

This is another verse that I frequently refer to, and with good reason. Confession is an outward way to declare what you believe in. It builds faith because faith comes by hearing. It also lets the Lord and the devil know where you stand. So speak aloud all the things you believe in. Repeat them over and over until they become a part of you.

Mark 16:17-18 And these signs will accompany those who believe: In my name they will drive out demons; they will speak in new tongues; they will pick up snakes with their hands; and when they drink deadly poison, it will not hurt them at all; they will place their hands on sick people, and they will get well.

As a believer, Jesus has given you the authority to drive out demons in His Name. You can use this authority during your pregnancy, labor, and delivery. You can command, in Jesus' Name, that your body functions properly. You can also command, in Jesus' Name, that you will not have certain pregnancy ailments or complications. And you can command the devil to flee from you. Jesus' Name holds incredible power.

The laying of hands is another powerful tool. Throughout your pregnancy, as the Lord leads, you can lay your hands over your abdomen and speak to your body. You can command your uterus to function properly. You can command the umbilical cord to be long enough and not wrapped around your baby's neck. You can command that the baby be born when it is fully ready. And if you've had specific complications in the past, speak to that area. You can speak to every part of your body and your baby. Jesus gives you this power.

So remain in faith. With the Lord, you are unmovable. You can enjoy a pregnancy free of all discomfort. You can enjoy a painless and complication-free labor and delivery. As a believer, you are under the Lord's authority. You are also heir to all of His promises.

The Child Within

Watching your belly grow and knowing what is going on inside of you is such a blessing. You are witnessing a miracle, firsthand, and your womb contains the work of God. It truly is a wondrous and awe-inspiring process. It is the creation of new life.

In God's eyes, when two people marry they become one. Similarly, cells from you and your husband have also joined as one. And this one cell contains everything needed to create another individual–your baby. Just like the Lord made Eve from one of Adam's ribs, He used a piece of each of you to create new life. What profound closeness this brings to a married couple–to join as one and be blessed with a life that is a part of both.

The following chart lists what is occurring in your belly throughout the pregnancy. Each month, look at this chart and visualize the precious baby inside of you. It is real–just as real as you and I. And when it is capable of surviving outside of your body, your body will gently push it into your loving arms.

Month of Gestation	Your Baby's Development
Month 1	Conception occurs as the sperm and egg join and become one. This one cell repeatedly divides as it travels from the fallopian tube to the uterus. The cells that are to be the placenta attach to the uterine wall. Meanwhile, amniotic fluid begins to develop, as well as the baby's central nervous system, a beating heart, lungs, and dark circles where the eyes will be. By the month's end, the baby is about the size of an apple seed.

Month 2	This month, the baby will begin developing internal ears, arms, hands, legs, a brain, major organs, the spinal cord, fingers with fingerprints, toes, and eyes with pigment. By the month's end, the baby is about the size of a grape.
Month 3	This month, the baby develops fingernails, toenails, external ears, internal and external sex organs, sperm in a boy, and ovaries and eggs in a girl. Blood now circulates through the umbilical cord, the baby's kidneys produce urine, and the baby's lungs can breathe amniotic fluid. By the month's end, the baby is about 3 ½ inches long and weighs approximately 2 ounces.
Month 4	This month, the baby's heartbeat can be easily heard. The baby also develops eyebrows and eyelashes. The baby is able to suck its thumb, kick, make facial expressions, and is sensitive to light. The baby is also covered in a fine hair called lanugo. By the month's end, the baby is about 5 inches long and weighs approximately 6 ounces.
Month 5	This month, the baby frequently exercises its muscles and you can feel it kick. The baby now has as many nerve cells as an adult, and has developed a sense of taste and smell. The baby is covered in a waxy substance called vernix. By the month's end, the baby is about 7 ½ inches long and weighs approximately 3/4 of a pound.
Month 6	This month, the baby has distinct patterns of sleeping and waking, and the ability to hiccup. By the month's end, the baby is about 9 inches long and weighs approximately 1 ½ pounds.
Month 7	This month, the baby has red, wrinkly skin, can react to sound, and has a digestive tract and lungs that are nearly mature. By the month's end, the baby is between 12 to 15 inches long and weighs approximately 2 ½ to 3 pounds.
Month 8	This month, the baby continues to gain weight and can possibly survive outside of the uterus. The baby may also be in the head-down position. By the month's end, the baby is about 19 inches long and weighs approximately 4 ½ pounds.

Month 9	This month, the baby continues to grow and gain weight. The vernix will mostly disappear, and the baby will develop meconium. By the month's end, the baby's position will change, it will drop into the pelvis, and the birth is imminent.

Chapter Four

For those of you who have been diligently handling your own prenatal care, the time has come to prepare for the labor and delivery. Again, research is the key. Learn what to expect and how to detect an emergency. Be prayerful about everything and strengthen your faith so that you can stand on it effortlessly.

Birthing Supplies

I have created a checklist of birthing supplies that I feel are necessary. Truthfully, as a friend once told me, the only necessity is a pregnant woman in labor. However, I am one to plan and the following supplies will help you to be prepared.

Birth Supply Checklist	
Item: **Waterproof Material** *Purpose:* To protect birthing area *Notes:* Try using a sheet of plastic or a shower curtain liner	

Item: **Absorbent Pads** (underpads) *Purpose:* To place over waterproof material to absorb blood and fluid *Notes:* Purchase online or at a medical supply store	
Item: **Old Blanket or Towel** *Purpose:* To wrap newborn in *Notes:* It may get stained	
Item: **Nasal Aspirator** *Purpose:* To suck fluid from baby's nose/mouth *Notes:* A nasal aspirator is often unnecessary	
Item: **Sterile White Shoe Laces or Cord Clamps** *Purpose:* To tie umbilical cord *Notes:* To sterilize, boil for 10 minutes, dry, and store in a sealed bag	
Item: **Sterile Scissors** *Purpose:* To cut umbilical cord *Notes:* To sterilize, boil for 10 minutes, dry, and store in a sealed bag	
Item: **Tincture of Shepard's Purse** *Purpose:* In case of hemorrhaging *Notes:* Take one dropper-full followed by a swig of water In an emergency, eating a portion of the placenta will stop hemorrhaging	
Item: **Tincture of Angelica** *Purpose:* To help uterus contract in the event of a retained placenta *Notes:* Take one dropper-full followed by a swig of water	
Item: **Bowl** *Purpose:* To examine and store placenta in *Notes:* Store placenta in refrigerator for emergency purposes	
Item: **Olive Oil** *Purpose:* For perineal massage to help prevent tears *Notes:* A white perineum indicates constricted blood vessels and is at risk for tearing	

Item: **First Aid Manual** *Purpose:* In case of an emergency *Notes:* It is important to be familiar with infant first aid *prior* to the delivery	
Labor Supplies Collect desired items to manage your labor (birth tub, birth ball, massage oils, etc.). Also collect important phone numbers (local hospital, family, friends), and if necessary, make childcare arrangements.	
Additional Supplies Be sure to have the necessary baby-care supplies at hand (diapers, clothes, bedding, etc.). It is also convenient to plan meals beforehand and delegate household chores. In addition, purchase an adequate supply of menstrual pads and nursing pads.	
Optional Supplies Baby Scale Ink (for hand and foot prints) Camera (with film/batteries if necessary) Video Camera (with blank tape/charged battery)	

Preparing for Labor

God specifically designed your body for the rigors of labor and delivery. You don't need anything other than faith and what He has equipped you with. Simply trust in the fact that you've been so wonderfully made!

However, there are non-drug techniques that you can use to aid in your comfort. Even if you are planning to trust in the Lord for a painless labor and delivery, these methods are still useful. They can help physically maintain your focus on having faith and not fear. These methods are also completely ethical by God's standards, unlike modern pain-control, and are safe and non-invasive.

Labor and Delivery Comfort Measures

Comfort Measure	Purpose/Benefit	How To Do It
Aromatherapy	To encourage relaxation	Lavender, sandalwood, lemon, and mint are all relaxing scents.
Birth Ball	To aid in relaxation To ease pain	While on your knees you can rest your upper body on the birth ball. Or, you can sit on it and sway your body during a contraction.
Counter-Pressure	To ease back pain	Have somebody press steadily on your lower back in different locations to see which is most effective.
Double Hip Squeeze	To ease back pain	While leaning forward on a bed or other sturdy object, have somebody firmly press each hip inward.
Heat and Cold	To ease pain	Either use a hot towel or water bottle on your lower back to relieve pain. A warm compress can be used on your perineum. Cold packs can relieve pain from hemorrhoids or stitches.
Hydrotherapy	To ease pain Known as the "midwives epidural"	Take a bath or shower for as long as it feels beneficial. You *can* bathe with ruptured membranes.

Knee Press	To relieve back pressure	Sit upright in a chair and have somebody cup their hands over your knees and gently press toward your back.
Massage	To ease pain	Gentle strokes can be reassuring between contractions while more intense massaging can help ease pain.
Movement and Position Change	To ease pain To help labor progress	Change your position every half hour.
Music	To aid in relaxation	Choose music that creates a relaxing environment. There are labor CD's created specifically for this purpose.
Relaxation	To feel less pain by allowing your body to go limp	Relax every muscle from your head to your toes, concentrating on one muscle at a time. Relaxation is the goal of most comfort measures.
TENS (Transcutaneous Electrical Nerve Stimulation)	To diminish the awareness of pain	Four flexible pads are connected by wires to a small battery-operated generator of electrical impulses. The pads adhere to your skin near your lower spine. During a contraction, you turn up two dials until you feel enough of a sensation to distract you from your pain.

I have excluded a few common relaxation techniques due to being leery of their roots. These include acupressure, hypnosis, visualization, and attention focusing. Most of these are new-age or of questionable origin, and clearly not appropriate for this book.

Besides the above chart, there are other ways to make labor more comfortable, such as dim lighting and favorite foods and beverages. If you are delivering away from home, you may also like to bring your pillow, a familiar blanket, or similar items.

Doula Care

Another invaluable addition to any labor and delivery is the presence of a *Doula*. A Doula is a female birth assistant. She is well-trained, experienced, and will provide continuous physical, emotional, and informational support. She is truly an indispensable asset.

With a Doula by your side, you will experience a shorter labor, fewer complications, less discomfort, less postpartum depression, and a greater satisfaction with your birth experience. Really, she is a gentle hand and a soft, encouraging voice to guide you through a long and trying process.

I, myself, have never had the experience or the pleasure of being assisted by a Doula. It wasn't until I became a Doula-in-training and attended my first birth that I realized what an impact one can truly have. It convinced me that every woman should have one.

I entered my first labor well-learned in book knowledge and in my own experiences. Although the training was beneficial, it was me, as a woman, which made the greatest impact. I didn't suddenly develop superpowers that could diminish pain and speed through time. Instead, I became a part of the woman's labor. I stayed by her side from the beginning of intensity to the very end. I reassured her that everything was going exactly as it should. I reminded her to breathe, to change position, and to stay focused on the end result–her baby. I reassured her that she was doing a wonderful job and that the end was near. Most important, I was there for her 100%. I was awake, alert, and within arms reach. I massaged her and comforted her. And I was blessed to witness the birth of her beautiful son.

During the labor, I followed my instincts and did what I felt I needed to do to be supportive of her in every way. It wasn't until afterwards that I truly realized what an impact I had. Never before, in my entire life, was I ever showered in so many sincere and heartfelt compliments. I made a difference in her life, and she was so appreciative. She even stated that she couldn't have done it without me. I know, just as she knows, that she could have. But my presence made it easier. My voice and touch carried her through. It still brings tears to my eyes just thinking about the experience. It makes me wish that I had that support at my own births.

Now don't misunderstand me. Husbands do make wonderful birth partners. However, there is something so natural about being supported by another woman–an experienced woman. In addition, it helps the husband. It allows him to rest when his wife rests. It allows him to support her at a level he feels comfortable. And it doesn't pressure him to feel that he should know exactly what to do to help ease her discomfort. He can be who he is, and in labor, that is exactly what the mother needs.

Regardless of where you plan to deliver–at home, in a birthing center, or in a hospital, consider what a Doula could do for you.

Preparing for Birth

The following chart lists exercises that you can practice beforehand to prepare your body for the labor and delivery. You should begin these exercises around mid-pregnancy, or sooner if possible.

Birth Preparation Exercises

Exercise	Purpose/Benefit	How To Do It
Kegels	Strengthens pelvic muscles Helps in the pushing stage Helps baby to rotate and descend	*Pelvic Floor Toning:* Contract the muscles of your pelvic floor as if you were trying to keep from urinating. Do some quick contractions and hold others for up to thirty seconds (Super Kegels). *Pelvic Floor Bulging:* Do this after a Super Kegel. Let go of the contraction and bulge your pelvic floor by gently straining as you would to pass out the last few drops of urine. End by contracting, then relaxing, the pelvic floor. Repeat a few times per day.
Pelvic Rock	Improves circulation Relieves low back pain Strengthens abdominal muscles Positions baby favorably	Get down on your hands and knees with your back straight, not sagging. Tuck your bottom under, feeling the tightening of your abdominal muscles and some arching and stretching in your lower back. Hold this position for a few seconds, then return to the original position. Repeat five or more times per day.
Perineal Massage	Prepares perineum to stretch Reduces need for episiotomy Reduces likeliness of tearing	Wash your hands and lubricate them with olive oil. Place two fingers well inside your vagina and rotate them in opposite directions upward along the sides and back to the center while pulling outward gently. Begin practicing four to six weeks before your due date and repeat for three to five minutes.

Squats	Helps baby to descend	Stand with your legs apart and your feet flat on the floor. Lower yourself into a squatting position and hold it for thirty seconds to one minute. Repeat five to ten times per day.

Signs of Labor

Along with faith, knowing what to expect will help the labor and delivery go more smoothly. Fear thrives on lack of faith and ignorance. It is important to meditate on God's Word night and day, to desire to know His ways, and to not doubt Him. Second to that, educate yourself on the process that your body will be going through. This way, the enemy will not be given a stronghold.

The signs of labor can be split into three categories: Potential signs, preliminary signs, and positive signs.

Potential Signs	Dull backache Recurring soft bowel movements Menstrual-type cramps "Nesting"–a sudden burst of energy
Preliminary Signs	Blood-tinged mucus–"the show" Hind leak–a gush or trickle of water followed by little else Non-progressing contractions Dropping or lightening
Positive Signs	Regular contractions Spontaneous rupture of the membranes

Potential Signs

The potential signs of labor are often difficult to detect. In the final trimester, backache is a common complaint, whether labor is impending or not. However, this type of backache is different. It tends to be quite consistent and an annoyance. You may even notice it following an on and off pattern, similar to contractions. A warm bath can ease the discomfort, but may thwart the onset of labor.

Soft bowel movements are another unclear indication, but do show that the time is near. It is usually caused by a rise in hormones, and helps by clearing more space for the baby's passage. Many women will experience soft bowel movements throughout the entire labor.

The menstrual-type discomfort you may experience is often your earliest contractions. It may come and go, and be more intense at times. This discomfort will eventually strengthen and turn into highly productive contractions. Until then, this is a perfect opportunity to practice relaxation.

Nesting may be the most difficult sign to detect. Some women experience it, and others don't. However, it occurs often enough that it is considered a common sign that labor is impending.

Nesting can manifest itself in different ways. Some women experience a sudden burst of energy. They may want to organize, cook, clean, or do the final birth preparations. Other women feel anxious and eager to prepare the house for the baby. They may sift through clothing, wash diapers, install the car seat, prepare the basinet, or pack the diaper bag. And many women simply feel restless. Either way, nesting usually proves to be productive and is completely harmless.

Preliminary Signs

The preliminary signs of labor are more noticeable and definitely indicate that labor is on its way. You may begin losing your mucus plug, also known as the *bloody show*, a week or so before labor begins. Some women don't begin losing it until labor is well established. Be forewarned, however, that the term *mucus plug* is a little deceiving. This plug isn't a single, solid piece of mucus, as the term may suggest. Instead, it comes in globs of blood-tinged mucus discharge and can continue throughout the labor.

Other women lose a bit of their amniotic fluid. If you experience a single gush followed by nothing else, then it is probably just a leak. If your bag of waters actually breaks, you will experience an ongoing trickle.

Non-progressing contractions have been unnoticeably occurring throughout much of your pregnancy. But as the end is in sight, they become stronger and more apparent. These contractions are usually unorganized and come and go at random. They may seem to progress for a few minutes, then suddenly stop. They may feel quite strong for hours, and then gradually dissipate. Just remember that your body is warming up.

Dropping and lightening are terms used for when the mother feels the baby descend–or drop lower into her abdomen. This usually does not cause dilation, but the mother may experience sensations that are similar to contractions. These sensations are caused by the stretching of the lower part of the uterus.

Positive Signs

Contractions are the most common way that labor begins. They may be irregular at first, but if they progress, you know that labor has begun. Progressing contractions become longer and stronger, with shorter breaks in between. You can time them to see if they are actually progressing or not.

Some women have strong and rapidly progressing contractions right from the start. Other women begin very slowly and gradually build intensity. But once these contractions are regular, you can expect them to escalate and eventually aid in the birth of your precious baby.

The most positive and instant sign that labor has begun is if your membranes rupture. This is also known as your bag of waters breaking. It will continually trickle and may be mistaken for urine. The water, or amniotic fluid, should be clear without a foul odor. If it is colored, this means that your baby has passed meconium, or in other words, a bowel movement. If under the care of a midwife, you will want to contact her immediately and note the time and the color of the fluid.

Meconium-stained amniotic fluid may appear alarming, and it can pose complications, but isn't likely to. And it isn't a contradiction to a home-birth. Many babies are born with dense meconium and have no further problems. The concern is if the baby inhales this substance. You must evaluate the situation after the birth, and if concerned, have it checked out.

The Labor and Delivery Process

During labor, your body will be going through many changes, and you will be feeling numerous sensations. The most noticeable will be the vigorous contractions of your uterus. The uterus, after all, is the largest and strongest muscle in the female body.

In active labor, the contractions will be intense and it is important to remain relaxed. Your uterus is working toward squeezing the baby out. However, when you tense your muscles, you are inadvertently holding the baby in. *These opposite forces will cause pain.*

For those of you with a previous Cesarean, try not to be overly concerned with uterine rupture. It is highly unlikely to occur, despite popular belief. But as a safety precaution, be aware of the warning signs, such as a hard, boardlike uterus.

Another thing that will be occurring during labor is the

softening, thinning, and opening of your cervix. The cervix begins at about 1 ½ inches in length and pointing toward your back. It then gradually moves forward and becomes paper thin. This thinning is measured in two ways: Centimeters and percentages.

Centimeters:

Three to four centimeters means that no thinning has occurred.
Two centimeters means that the cervix has thinned about half way.
Less than one centimeter means the cervix is almost paper-thin.

Percentages:

Zero percent means that no thinning has occurred (3-4 centimeters).
Fifty percent means that the cervix is thinned half way (2 centimeters).
One-hundred percent means the cervix is paper-thin (less than 1 centimeter).

One important thing to note is that cervical thinning is not the same thing as cervical dilation. Yet cervical dilation is also measured in centimeters. The total cervical dilation will be approximately ten centimeters.

As your labor progresses, your baby will move lower in your abdomen. Before sliding through your birth canal, his or her head will rotate to make an easier fit. It may even mold to an elongated shape. This is usually temporary and will even out on its own.

The descent of your baby as it moves through your body is measured in terms of *station*. It ranges from minus four to plus four. The negative numbers indicate how many centimeters the baby is above your pelvis. The positive numbers indicate how close the baby is to being born. Zero station would indicate that the baby is at your mid-pelvis.

The following chart lists the stages of labor and delivery. Although the terminology is unimportant, knowing the gist of things is. If you know how labor works, you will be able to detect which part you are in and what to expect.

Labor and Delivery: What To Expect

Stage	Sub-Stage (if applicable)	Duration	Progress/ What To Expect
Pre-Labor		On and off for hours or days	Cervix softens, thins, and moves forward. Uterus contracts in preparation for labor.
First: Dilation Stage	Early Labor	Lasts a few hours to 20 hours	Cervix continues to thin and dilates from 0 to 5 centimeters You may feel menstrual-like cramping, backache, and have soft bowel movements
	Active Labor	Lasts ½ to 6 hours	Cervix dilates from 5 to 8 centimeters Contractions become intense and painful Contractions last 60 seconds or more Contractions come every 4 minutes or less You may feel aching in your back or legs
	Transition Phase	Lasts 10 to 60 minutes	Cervix dilates from 8 to 10 centimeters Contractions are long and painful with little break in between Baby may begin descending and causing pressure You may feel restless, tense, and overwhelmed You may want to give up You may tremble and vomit You may have hot or cold flashes You may feel shaky

Second: Birthing Stage	Resting Phase	Lasts 0 to 20 minutes	Baby's head may be in birth canal Cervix is fully dilated You may become clear-headed and optimistic. Contractions may stop or slow down
	Descent Phase	Lasts 10 minutes to 2 ½ hours	Strong contraction resume Baby moves down the birth canal The urge to push becomes strong and unavoidable
	Crowning and Birth Phase	Lasts 1 to 20 minutes	Birth of the head is imminent You may feel intense burning in your vagina Baby's head emerges and rotates Baby's shoulders and the rest of the body are born
Third: Placental Stage		Lasts 5 minutes to 2 hours	You may be very shaky Your uterus cramps Your placenta separates from the uterine wall Your placenta is delivered

If you are planning to deliver in a hospital, whether by choice or necessity, it is a good idea to be familiar with common procedures. This way, they won't seem so frightening and you will be able to make informed decisions of what you will and will not allow. You do have a choice!

And finally, at the risk of being repetitive, I can not stress enough the importance of faith. Build your faith so that it is immoveable. Let it be a fortress where you can find peace, rest, and confidence. May God be with you as you embark on this miraculous and profound journey.

Your Newborn

Immediately after the birth, regardless of how long and tiring it may have been, you will be awake, alert, and ready to meet your baby. However, your baby may not be as you had expected. He or she may be red, swollen, covered in *vernix*, or covered in a soft, downy hair, known as *lanugo*. A *postmature* baby, which is a baby born after his or her due date, may have peeling skin. All of these attributes are normal and will resolve on their own. The picture-perfect newborn that many mothers visualize will emerge within a few days. What you are witnessing is the beautiful phenomenon of life in the raw.

As soon as your baby is born, lay him or her directly on your belly, skin to skin, and cover the two of you in a blanket. This will help to retain heat and promote mother/infant bonding. There is no need to bathe your baby at this point. If he or she is soiled with blood, meconium, or other birth debris, gently wipe it off with a warm, damp cloth. If *vernix* is present, which is a waxy substance, simply massage it into your baby's skin.

After you and your newborn have had a few moments to rest and become acquainted, it is time to initiate your first breast-feeding experience. Most babies will be eager to nurse immediately and there is no need to delay. *The sooner you nurse your baby, the better.* This can be accomplished prior to the delivery of the placenta and the cutting of the cord.

At birth, the umbilical cord will be bluish-purple and pulsating. *Special care should be taken to avoid tugging on it.* Once the cord becomes thin and white, it is then safe to tie and cut it. However, there is no harm in delaying this step for as long as you'd like.

When you are ready, simply tie a sterile shoe lace (or use a cord clamp) about six to twelve inches from your baby's body, and another about one inch from that. Cut between the ties (or clamps.)

When the placenta is ready to be expelled, your uterus will begin contracting. Gently push out the placenta. It is a simple and painless process. The placenta should be stored in a container until it can be examined for completeness.

For more information on birth and your newborn baby, see Birth: A Closer Look, found in Chapter Seven.

Postpartum

After the delivery of your baby and placenta, you should nurse your baby to encourage your uterus to contract. This can also be accomplished by massaging your uterus through your belly. A soft and relaxed uterus will bleed too heavily, so it is important to ensure that it is tightening. A tightened uterus will feel like a softball. Your postpartum bleeding will last for approximately two to six weeks, sometimes longer.

When your baby nurses, you will most likely experience after-pains. Although uncomfortable, it is a good indication that your uterus is contracting and all is well. Try relaxing through the pains just as you did in labor.

If your perineum is sore or swollen, ice packs or baths can help ease the discomfort. Making a tea out of ginger may also prove to be beneficial in easing the pains.

Chapter Five

B efore the arrival of your little blessing, you will want to have decided a few important things. How do you plan to feed your baby (as if that was really a question!)? Are you going to vaccinate? Have you thought of alternatives to disposable diapers? Where is the baby going to sleep? Do you plan to work or stay at home? And a few thoughts that come to mind while looking into the near future: Discipline, entertainment, and schooling.

Breast-Feeding

Isaiah 49:15 Can a mother forget the baby at her breast and have no compassion on the child she has borne? . . .

In biblical times and throughout most of history, breast-feeding was the only choice. It was also a logical, God-honoring practice. In the rare case that a woman couldn't nurse her baby, another woman would do it for her. This way, the baby would still have all the benefits of breast-feeding. But what are the benefits? And what happens when we stray from God's original plan?

To begin, human breast milk contains *all* of the nutrients and substances that a baby needs. It is pure, easy to digest, and provides essential antibodies to protect against illness. It even changes as the baby's needs change, being nutritionally-complete for all levels of development. And unlike formula, human breast milk seldom causes allergies or other physical problems. It is truly the world's perfect food.

Due to false advertising, many unsuspecting parents have been fooled into believing that formula is comparable to breast milk. In *no* way is this true! For one thing, scientists don't even know exactly what is in breast milk, which makes it *impossible* to duplicate. With that said, *all* formula-fed infants are lacking essential substances that can only be found in breast milk.

Did you know that at birth your baby's brain is not fully developed? Once the developmental process ends, around age three, brain cells may die, yet no new brain cells will grow. So it is crucial for your baby to receive the proper nutrition in the early months. Formula *cannot* support the proper growth of a baby's brain. *Only* breast milk can. It is a living substance and unmatchable.

Breast-feeding not only has benefits for your baby, but for you as well. It helps you to heal after childbirth, to return to your pre-pregnancy weight, and prevents certain types of cancer. More than these, it promotes true mother/infant bonding, which is something that formula-feeding mothers often lack.

Besides health reasons, breast-feeding is the motherly and womanly thing to do. It is also convenient–no heating, sterilizing, or stirring. It allows your baby to be with you, skin to skin, while you soothe him or her with what comes naturally. And it makes no sense–morally or physically–to withhold the only thing your newborn wants and needs–you.

As for formula companies, their sole interest is to make money. They do not care about your baby or the rising health crisis in the United States which is largely due to formula consumption.

They portray formula as the modern and socially-acceptable way of feeding a baby. At one time or another, we are all led astray by false advertising. Quite often, we are derailed by our own good-intentioned family members.

If you think about it logically, how safe can it be to rely on a canister of powder or a pre-made shake to fulfill a baby's dietary needs? It isn't. Formula is a created substance–a *formula*–and artificial in every way. Only animals should be fed in such a rudimentary manner, not human babies!

From a similar perspective, what competent individual would feed a toddler the same pre-packaged food, meal after meal, day after day? No one! That would be child-neglect. So why is this practice viewed as normal and acceptable for a newborn baby? Is a newborn less-than-human? Does a newborn need less than an older child? Absolutely not! They need more–they need the living food that can only be found in their mother's breasts.

Breast-feeding, which is becoming a lost art, can be difficult and awkward in the early days. However, choosing to rely on formula isn't the answer. It takes patience and support. Not only do you have to learn to breast-feed, but your baby does also.

When it comes to breast-feeding, pray to the Lord and He will make your efforts successful. Pretend that there isn't an alternative–there isn't a safe one, anyway. And work at it until it becomes easier. It is really worth it–for you, your baby, and the women around you.

Once your baby is born, he or she will be ready to nurse immediately–even before the umbilical cord is cut. *The sooner your baby latches on, the better.* In my opinion, the easiest and most elementary way to nurse a baby is in the *cradle hold*.

Sitting down, cradle your baby with your forearm, using the right arm to nurse on the right side and vice versa. Position your baby's body parallel to yours, with his or her head resting on the crook of your arm. Hold your breast with the opposite hand and insert your nipple into your baby's mouth. If your baby's mouth is closed, encourage him or her to open it by rubbing your nipple against his or her cheek, or allowing milk to fall on his or her lips.

Once latched on, be sure that your baby's bottom lip isn't tucked under. This will hurt your nipple and inhibit proper suction. You'll also want to make sure that your nipple is as far in your baby's mouth as possible.

Recognizing when your baby wants to nurse may take a little getting used to, but two clear indications are when they cry and their *rooting reflex*. The rooting reflex can be seen in a couple of ways.

First, while holding your baby, he or she may tilt their head toward the side looking for your breast. This motion shows that he or she wants to nurse.

Next, if you are holding your baby on your shoulder, he or she may *peck* at you. This is a more obvious display of the rooting reflex and again indicates that your baby wants to nurse.

In the early days, your baby may want to nurse all of the time. This is normal and does not mean that your baby is not getting enough milk. As long as you are nursing *on demand*, which is when your baby wants to, you can feel secure that he or she is getting enough.

On average, a newborn baby usually nurses every two hours. However, don't force any kind of rigid schedule. As long as your baby is nursing and content, all is well. Nurse as frequently as he or she wants. It isn't just about nursing, but bonding. And this first milk, called *colostrum*, is extremely important.

As alarming at it may be to new parents, it is not uncommon for a newborn baby to spit-up milk on a regular basis. This does not indicate an allergy or other underlying problem, but instead, an immature esophagus. The baby will grow out of this habit as he or she gets older.

Your baby's first bowel movements will be a very dark and sticky substance called *meconium*. Afterwards, your baby will begin having regular bowel movements. They should be very soft and either yellowish or greenish. Don't be alarmed at the texture or frequency. Your baby does not have diarrhea. It is perfectly normal.

Within a few days your milk will come in. You may become *engorged*, which is when your breasts are hard and tender due to an overabundance of milk. Frequent nursing will help until your milk-production regulates. If the baby is unable to latch on, try pumping first to reduce the pressure.

Between feedings you are likely to find the need to wear nursing pads. They fit into your bra and absorb any milk that may leak. Try to buy washable ones. They are more comfortable and better for you, your baby, and the environment.

One thing to watch out for is *mastitis,* which is a breast infection. If you notice any spots on your breasts that are reddened, hard, or particularly tender, you may have a clogged duct. This could turn into mastitis if it isn't resolved. Fortunately, there is an easy solution.

Using a damp, warm washcloth, or while bathing, firmly massage the tender area with your fingers, pressing toward your nipple. This will encourage the duct to clear and the milk flow to resume. After a few minutes, you should feel relief as the hardened area dissipates. Some women find that nursing the baby with the baby's chin pointing toward the clogged area will also help.

Another aspect of breast-feeding that is worth mentioning is the *letdown reflex*. While your baby first nurses, he or she will work quite vigorously to get the milk out. Then suddenly, letdown occurs and your baby may even choke on the overabundance. This is normal and your baby will get used to it.

If you are concerned about an inadequate milk supply, the most important thing that you can do is to consume a health-promoting diet. There are also herbs that help, such as blessed thistle and nettle leaf, which both encourage abundant milk production. You can create your own tea, or purchase a pre-packaged version at a natural food store.

Keep in mind, however, that a lack of breast milk is highly unlikely. Even malnourished women in poorer countries are able to produce adequate milk for their young. This is the Lord's way of providing a healthy beginning for each and every baby.

Some babies will stop nursing, or *wean* themselves, within the first year of life. This is fine as long as the baby initiated it. Others will continue to nurse well into their second, third, fourth, or even fifth year of life. This *is* normal and not a reason to wean! The baby will stop nursing when the time is right. And despite society's warped beliefs, there is nothing strange about nursing a toddler. What is strange is to see a human of any age drinking *cow's* breast milk. Talk about needing to be weaned!

Despite what others may say, even doctors, there is absolutely *no* need to give your baby formula, water, or anything other than your breast milk. Your baby can live exclusively off of your breast milk for six months, or even longer, *without* supplementation. Wait until he or she indicates the readiness to try other things. Then you may feed them according to their interest and ability.

Nursing is often challenging, but mostly because of the uneducated views of others. People often create all sorts of problems, almost as if they hope that you fail. They may say that the baby isn't getting enough, your breasts are too large or too small, you have inverted nipples, your baby is dehydrated, and so on. Try not to listen or fall victim to their uneducated views. Instead, rely on the instincts that the Lord gave you and know that you are using your breasts as He intended.

Although I could provide you with a wealth of nursing knowledge, I won't. You shouldn't worry about positions, techniques, alternative methods, and pumping. Instead, concentrate on what comes naturally. Rely on your instincts, and if unsure, rely on another experienced woman for guidance. If no help is available, read books specifically dedicated to breast-feeding.

Whether you have small breasts, large breasts, flat nipples, or a fussy baby, none of that matters. What matters is that you look at breast-feeding as your only choice. *It will work if you make it work.* It is the best possible food for your growing baby, and your baby does deserve the best. Why rob your baby of the one God-given thing that gives him or her a healthy and secure beginning?

Vaccinations

When it comes to vaccinations, most parents are compliant with their doctor's recommendation. They seldom question the doctor's motives, often because they feel inadequate to make an informed decision of their own. However, the decision to vaccinate isn't one to take lightly. It is a life or death decision–one that cannot be reversed. Although parents are bound to make mistakes, this is one mistake that they cannot afford.

Adverse vaccine reactions may occur immediately upon exposure, or be delayed for days, weeks, months, and even years. These adverse effects include a weakened immune system, fever, rash, asthma, shock, deafness, convulsions, seizures, paralysis, mental retardation, learning disabilities, epilepsy, behavioral disorders, arthritis, brain damage, and even death. The immunized child is also put at risk of contracting the vaccinated disease itself–something that would otherwise be improbable. Considering that these adverse reactions aren't uncommon, each parent must earnestly ask themselves: Is the risk worth taking?

Each year, thousands of unsuspecting parents inject their children with toxins such as aluminum, thimerosal (mercury), and formaldehyde. They do not grasp the underlying danger, and naively assume that they are doing the right thing. Yet realistically, they are compromising their child's very life. And for what?

Some diseases that children are vaccinated against don't even exist anymore. They were not eradicated by vaccinations, as the vaccine industry would like for you to believe, but by their own life process. These diseases disappeared around the globe, even in countries that did not vaccinate. So why endanger a child's life for an unlikely threat?

Today, there are safer alternatives to traditional vaccinations–ones that contain minimal toxins. However, this issue goes deeper than the mere avoidance of toxic chemicals. As believers, we must obey our Creator and His rules for life–the Bible.

Leviticus 17:10-12 Any Israelite or any alien living among them who eats any blood–I will set my face against that person who eats blood and will cut him off from his people. For the life of a creature is in the blood, and I have given it to you to make atonement for yourselves on the alter; it is the blood that makes atonement for one's life. Therefore I say to the Israelites, "None of you may eat blood, nor may an alien living among you eat blood."

Acts 15:20 Instead we should write to them, telling them to abstain from food polluted by idols, from sexual immorality, from the meat of strangled animals and from blood.

Vaccines are blood-products–that is, they are made out of blood. As the above verses clearly state, we are to abstain from blood, regardless of the form, because blood is the life of a creature. God commands that we are to avoid the intake of blood, and it is wise to heed to His instruction.

As the obedient children of God, it is clearly unacceptable to inject our children with blood. It is also unacceptable to risk their lives *just in case* they may come into contact with something. Instead, we must rely on the Lord and know that good health ultimately comes from Him alone.

Diapering

As a natural mother, you may or may not have considered alternatives to disposable diapers. Within the web of baby-care options, this one often falls last on the list. But with so many wonderful and convenient alternatives, it is definitely worth looking into.

Regular disposable diapers aren't as innocent as they appear. They contain highly toxic substances that are absorbed by a baby's skin. These substances, in the form of gel-like beads, often enter a little girl's vagina. One can only imagine the negative effects, ranging from infertility to cancer.

As for little boys, disposable diapers are efficient insulators, resulting in the overheating of their testicles. It is common knowledge that long periods of overheating result in decreased fertility. Although this is not an issue now, these effects are long-term and may cause fertility issues in the future.

Besides the direct health risks, disposable diapers pose other problems. They are wasteful, environmentally unfriendly, and unsanitary. Lingering in landfills, these dirty diapers are full of disease-infested fecal matter, including diseases that the child has been recently vaccinated against. These diseases, along with the diaper's own toxins, are absorbed into the ground, or run off into the fields and streams.

Natural food stores do carry a safer alternative to your average disposable diaper. They still have the convenience of the disposables, without the toxicity. But there is still a better option–cloth!

Cloth diapers aren't what they used to be. There is no longer a need for diaper pins or plastic pants, unless that's the method you choose. There are many brands, colors, patterns, styles, and sizes. Shopping for diapers has never been so fun!

Using cloth diapers have absolutely *no* health risks for your baby or the environment. This alone is reason enough to use them, but they are also more sanitary. Once your baby has a bowel movement, toss the fecal matter into the toilet and flush. Then the soiled diaper sits in a sealed container (diaper pail) until wash day.

Cloth diapers are affordable, although they do require a bit more money up front. Once purchased, they will last and last. Depending on the brand, they may be used for multiple children.

You can purchase cloth diapers that are pre-folded, all-in-one, or ones with different style covers that you place absorbent material within. They come with snaps, hooks, Velcro, and some still have pins. It all depends on what you are looking for, and the options seem endless. It is truly a wonderful, God-honoring alternative, and I am grateful that they are so easy to come by. Plus, if you are handy on the sewing machine, you can even make your own.

When washing cloth diapers, try using natural laundry products. Definitely avoid bleach and other chemicals. Having a healthy child is more important than your whites being snow-white. If interested, try using baking soda or vinegar instead. Also, avoid fabric softeners and dryer sheets. They will leave a residue that can irritate your baby's skin.

As for baby-wipes, try making your own. Chemical-free paper towels can be cut or folded into the desired size, placed in a sealable container, and dampened with a homemade solution.

To create your own wipe solution, simply mix water with a bit of natural liquid soap, such as organic baby body wash. Experiment to find the desired moisture level. In addition, there are many things you can add to this wipe solution, such as herbs, to help treat and prevent diaper rash.

For those of you who are environmentally-conscious, wash cloths make excellent reusable wipes. Simply dampen the cloth under the faucet and wipe. If you are on an outing where water is not available, put a few wash cloths in a sealable container with your own wipe solution. Just be sure to have a bag to toss the soiled cloths in. When finished, toss the cloths in the diaper pail until wash day.

While diligently taking care of your child's diapering needs, it is wise to also think of yourself. Menstrual products contain many of the same toxins found in disposable diapers and are also environmentally unfriendly. But just like your child, you also have safe alternatives. From cloth menstrual pads, to natural tampons and tampon-type products, there are so many options. Choosing to use these products will make you feel better about yourself and the environment. Sometimes Mommy needs a little pampering too!

Sleeping

Sleep, or the lack of it, is an issue for most new parents. It is a much talked about subject, rendering a heap of sleep strategies that are as varied as the babies themselves. Many parents will desperately skip from one failed strategy to another, only to be left wondering why *their* baby is so difficult.

At this point, parents often conclude that something must be wrong with their baby. They may speculate colic, gas, or some other discomfort. What they fail to realize is that a baby isn't born with the ability to put itself to sleep. It is an acquired skill, and until it is mastered, most babies do need help in one form or another. Some need more help than others.

Unfortunately, as most books will not tell you, no single sleep strategy will work for every baby. Different babies have different needs. Because of this, each parent needs to act accordingly, providing precisely what their baby needs to drift into dreamland.

Some "experts" say that a baby should be left alone to *cry it out*. They claim that the baby will learn to self-soothe, and that any other sleep method, such as rocking the baby, will spoil the child and instill bad sleep habits. This theory is simply not true!

First, it is *impossible* to spoil a newborn baby. *A baby's wants are its needs.* Furthermore, if spoiling were possible, the damage would have already been done in the womb. Your womb was a place where your baby's needs were instantly met even before your baby needed them. There was no such thing as being too hot or too cold, hungry or thirsty, overtired or overstimulated. Your baby was constantly rocked, cuddled, and carried. Realistically speaking, no place outside of the womb could compete!

Second, newborn babies are not equipped to deal with abandonment, which is what a parent is doing when they allow their baby to cry it out. When abandonment occurs, the baby's defense mechanism is triggered, causing the baby to mentally shut-down. This act of survival expends so much of the baby's energy that the baby will lack the sufficient means to even develop properly.

In our society, we have been misled into believing that independence can be taught–and, the sooner the better. However, independence is a trait that is gradually acquired through maturity and life experience. It cannot be taught to anyone, and especially not to a newborn baby. There is no other human more dependent than a newborn, and to try to force independence is not only absurd, but often inhumane.

Even so, the average American mother takes pride in "teaching" her baby to sleep alone at an early age. It is considered a great feat, and once accomplished, she feels competent not only as a mother, but as a woman. But is overcoming this challenge something to take pride in?

It doesn't take an expert to realize that forcing a baby to cry it out is wrong. It takes a mother. Allowing a baby to cry it out is heart-wrenching, and rightfully so. God specifically designed a newborn baby's cry to demand the attention that he or she needs. It is a sound that should never be ignored.

Other "experts" feel that you must choose a specific method

of putting your baby to sleep–the same method that you plan to use forever and ever. This is based on the premise that babies need predictability, and that it is very difficult to teach a child a new way to drift off to sleep.

Sure, babies do need predictability. They need to know that someone will comfort them when they cry. They need to know that they'll be fed when they are hungry, or changed when they are wet. However, a change in sleep habits is not a life-altering event. Babies are forever changing, and you must learn to change as they do. Just because you decide to rock your baby to sleep now does not mean that you will be rocking them to sleep five years from now.

To their mother's delight, some babies are quite content to sleep alone. They can be put in a bassinet, eyes wide open, and peacefully drift off without a single twitch or cry. As desirable of a characteristic as this may be, it is the exception, not the rule.

For the first two weeks or so of your baby's life, he or she will sleep easily. Matter of fact, that is all he or she will be doing, with the exception of eating and eliminating.

However, around two to three weeks of age, your baby will begin having set periods of awake and asleep time. Maybe he or she will want to nurse to sleep. Maybe he or she will want to be rocked or carried to sleep. Or maybe it won't be that simple.

Some babies have a much more difficult time drifting off to sleep than others. And, since your baby does not know how to fall asleep, you will have to help him or her. Your finicky baby will most likely respond positively to stimuli that reminds him or her of their first "home," your womb.

To begin, your womb wasn't a quiet place. It was full of swishing and pulsating sounds. It wasn't a still place either. Your baby was rocked, bumped, and jiggled. So, as you can imagine, it would be difficult for your baby to fall asleep in the still, quiet environment that so many parents try to produce.

Most babies don't mind constant noise, whether it be a radio, vacuum cleaner, or hair dryer. It is comforting to them. Even more comforting, and nearly irresistible to fight, is movement. Not soft, gentle movements, but fairly large, bumpy movements.

Here's a bit of sleep history with my own three children. I've included it to show just how different babies can be–even within the same family.

My first child, Natalia, was easy to please. I didn't need to rock her, walk with her, or nurse her incessantly. Instead, she was simply content to be held. I could hold her on my lap and watch the television. I could hold her over my shoulder and listen to the radio. She'd sleep on my chest at night, and lay in my lap, quiet as a mouse, while I'd eat.

As she grew older, she learned to self-soothe by sucking on two of her fingers. She seemed to always try to get her hands in her mouth from as early on as I can remember, but didn't actually get the hang of it until she was about five months old. She then earned the nickname "Two-fingered Tali."

A couple of months later we moved, and this disrupted her sleep habits. She was still content to be held and suck on her fingers, but laying her down to nap was impossible. I'd lay with her and she'd fuss and cry. Once asleep, she'd be easily awoken by any noise. Nighttime wasn't pleasant either.

Those times were frustrating, but very short lived. During nap time one day, Natalia was fussing and grabbed a hold of my hair. She wrapped it around her two fingers, put her fingers in her mouth, and fell fast asleep.

From that point on, my hair, or "hairy," as we call it, was a lifesaver. It didn't matter where we were, what time it was, or how noisy it was. As long as my daughter had her two fingers and my hair, she was so quiet and content. It always amused our family and friends.

Now, at five years of age, she still sucks on her fingers but twirls her own hair. She falls asleep instantly and can sleep through anything. She slept in our bed for the first few years of her life, and has now happily moved to her own bed.

My second child, Cheyenne, was nicknamed "Cry-anne" very early on. She seemed grumpy from the day she was born, and it was difficult to make her happy. Well–it was difficult to make her happy without nursing.

During the first week of Cheyenne's life she realized how much she loved nursing, or "nummies," as we call it, and she didn't want to live without it. It took me a few days to realize that the only way I would get any sleep at night was if I nursed her lying down. As long as she was latched on, she was content. She could just nurse and nurse and nurse.

Nap time was never very challenging. She'd become tired, I'd nurse her, and then I'd transfer her to bed. She'd sleep for a reasonable amount of time, awake, and nurse. We'd go through that all day long.

As she grew older, she never grew out of loving nummies. I felt differently. I didn't mind nursing her during the day, but at age two, she was still waking me up in the middle of the night for one feeding. I'd awake to find her face very close to mine and a soft, sweet voice saying, "Mommy, may I please have nummies?"

Sometime before her third birthday, I weaned her of her nighttime nummies. She cried in the beginning, but got over it very quickly. Matter of fact, she soon discontinued nummies all together.

In hindsight, I realized that Cheyenne didn't have her own self-soothing technique like her older sister, Natalia. She relied on me to pacify herself.

Now, at age three, she occasionally awakes during the night for a bit of reassurance. For the most part, however, she sleeps well and in her own bed. Most importantly, she knows how to put herself to sleep.

By my third child, David, I assumed that sleeping would be a breeze. I was a seasoned mother of two very different children. I was older, wiser, and more patient.

To my surprise, however, David was the most difficult baby that I had ever encountered. He truly put my parenting skills to the test and gave a new meaning to sleep deprivation.

The first two weeks of his life were easy. He ate, slept, and soiled his diaper. It was a constant cycle. I thought that he was just the world's best baby.

By the time he reached three weeks of age, my perspective took a drastic turn for the worst. David would simply cry, and cry, and cry. Nothing I did would make a difference. I rocked him. I nursed him. I sung to him. I spent hours walking with him.

In the beginning, he'd sleep as long as I was moving. The moment I'd stop, his eyes would spring open and he'd begin to cry.

However, he eventually became so overtired that he wouldn't even sleep while I was walking with him. Instead, he'd scream with his eyes squeezed shut. If I was able to latch him on, he'd nurse for a moment, arch his back, and begin crying. He wasn't hungry, he was tired, and being fed only frustrated him further. The world's best baby turned into the world's worst baby overnight, and I felt so overwhelmed and isolated that I didn't know how to cope. I'd just cry right along with him.

Out of desperation, I began reading book after book on sleep. One said to let him cry until he fell asleep. I tried it, it was heart-wrenching, and I knew that it wasn't right. I then tried to lay him down, comfort him when he'd cry, then lay him back down again. He eventually became inconsolable. Truthfully, he cried more than he did anything else.

Finally, I made a breakthrough. I realized that he was only a baby and that he didn't know how to put himself to sleep. As his mother, I needed to find a way to simulate his first home–my womb–which was the only world he knew and found comfort in.

Through trial and error, I eventually discovered just what he needed to feel content enough to sleep.

First, I worked on positioning. I couldn't hold David horizontally because he associated it with nursing. I didn't want him to nurse. I wanted him to sleep. He also wasn't happy on my shoulder. Instead, he liked facing outward and observing his surroundings. There was an ornamental tree with lights on it that he showed a particular interest in.

Next, I put on an upbeat CD. It was something that I could dance to–a way to keep David jiggling just like he did in my belly. I played the CD at a comfortable volume that helped block out stray noises like my daughters' chattering.

And finally, I moved. David didn't like bouncing. David didn't like swaying. David didn't like rocking. However, I found a vigorous movement that pleased him. I'd sway back and forth, while simultaneously bouncing at the knees. It wasn't a gentle sway, but an energetic one.

I then put all of the elements together. First, I made sure that David had a full belly and was comfortable. I held him in my arms, facing outwards toward the ornamental tree. I then swayed and bounced to the CD. Within ten minutes, David was asleep. The atmosphere that I created was irresistible to him. He just melted in my arms.

Once asleep, I put David in his swing and kept the music playing. In the beginning, I felt guilty for allowing him to sleep in the swing. It seemed healthier to have him sleep in a bed. However, I realized that sometimes you just need to do what works.

For the next few weeks I put David to sleep in this same way. I always had the music, the tree for him to look at, and the movement. Sometimes I'd do my bouncy-sway movements, and at other times I'd downright dance. The more vigorous the movement, the faster he'd fall asleep. It normally took only three to five minutes, and then he'd sleep for an hour or more. I was finally able to comfort my baby and help him have an easy transition into my world. Plus, his newfound sleep turned him from being the world's grumpiest baby to the world's happiest baby.

To my delight, I eventually discovered that this sleep technique still worked even if a few of the elements were missing. One day, David awoke in the middle of my weekly grocery shopping and was about to have a total meltdown. I didn't have any music to play or a pretty tree for him to look at, but I still had me and movement. I assumed position and energetically bounced him from side to side. He fussed a bit, but my efforts ended in success! Although it wasn't easy, I completed my shopping with him asleep in one of my arms.

By the time he reached eight weeks of age, I decided to change how I put him to sleep. I felt that he was old enough to learn a new sleep method–one that was easier on my body. I began playing a CD of instrumental baby music, nursing him, placing him over my shoulder, and rocking in a rocking chair.

For the first few attempts, he cried for about fifteen minutes then fell asleep. Within a day or so, he'd whimper for a few minutes and fall asleep. Then, I'd transfer him to bed and he'd sleep for an hour. I did it! I finally had my baby sleeping in bed. That was a great accomplishment on my behalf.

Around sixteen weeks of age, David was still unable to put himself to sleep, which was becoming a problem. Nap time was simple, but nighttime wasn't so easy. He'd awake every two hours to nurse, and about once per night he needed to be rocked back to sleep. So again I made a change.

Instead of rocking David, I nursed him, put on his CD, and put him in bed next to me. The nursing and music alerted him to the fact that it was nap time, and he just needed to find a way to put himself to sleep.

He cried for a bit, which was sad to hear, but I reminded myself that he wasn't alone. I was right next to him. Soon enough, he discovered his hand and began to suck on his fist. Within a few minutes he was asleep.

I spent an entire day putting him down for naps in the same manner and the results were amazing. That very night, as he became cranky and ready for bed, I simply set him between my husband and I on our bed. He fussed a bit, and to my husband's surprise, David sucked on his fist, closed his eyes, and put himself to sleep. It was a very rewarding feeling as a parent.

That night, he only awoke a few times to nurse, and never needed to be rocked. If he was awake after a feeding, I simply set him back down and let him put himself to sleep.

As of now, my daughters are comfortably sleeping in their own room. In the beginning, they slept in bed with my husband and I. Then, we moved them to a bunk-bed within our room. Now, the bunk-bed is in their room. I've made small windows between our room and theirs so that if they ever need a bit of comfort, we are always in sight.

As for David, he is four months old and happily sleeping in bed with my husband and I. We will continue sleeping this way until he shows interest in sleeping alone.

Now years ago, it was common practice for a baby to sleep in bed with his or her parents, just as my family now does. No reasonable individual would expect anything else. And although a baby is still only a baby, today's parents have unrealistic expectations.

From the moment your baby is conceived, you are the only person he or she knows. Your baby finds comfort in your warmth, voice, rhythmic breathing, and every move. Your baby is lulled to sleep by these consistent, predictable, and soothing sounds and motions. All of his or her needs are met, and the only person your baby needs is you.

Upon birth, however, your baby is bombarded by sounds and

sensations that are foreign to him or her. For the first time your baby may feel cold, hungry, uncomfortable, or scared. Although he or she will eventually adjust, it does take time. Until then, you can soothe your baby with your touch, voice, motion, and breasts. He or she will need this constant comfort throughout the days *and* throughout the nights.

Having your baby sleep with you is often referred to as the *family bed*, or *co-sleeping*. The family bed can consist of only Mommy, Daddy, and baby, or children of all ages. There isn't a right or wrong. Instead, it is about nurturing those who need to be nurtured, and what works for your family. It is another extension of parent/child bonding.

If you like the idea of the family bed, but are afraid of hurting the baby during the night, there are precautions that you can take. Most importantly, you must know that rolling over the baby is highly unlikely if both parents are sober. Even so, there are alternatives.

First, there are cot-like beds that lie directly on top of your mattress. They have very low sides which can give your baby his or her own protective "nest" without inhibiting close parental contact. This is ideal if you would like to have the baby in bed with you, but are afraid of roll-overs.

Next, there are portable cribs and bassinets. Both of these can go directly against the side of your bed and often have a side panel that folds down so that the baby is in arm's reach. If you want your baby to be close, but not in bed, this option is ideal.

For squirmy toddlers, you may want to consider a simple bed-rail to help prevent falls. A bed-rail can also be used for newborns, but caution must be taken to ensure that your baby doesn't become pinched between the rail and your mattress.

And some children are simply content to be in your bedroom, not necessarily your bed. If you have the adequate space, try to fit a separate bed, or bunk-bed, for your toddler or older children. It is always safer for families to sleep together, especially in the event of an emergency.

Whatever method you use, know that co-sleeping is truly a wonderful experience. Babies are only babies once. Spend as much time as you can–awake or asleep–with your little blessing. You will develop a bond that can never be broken, and a trust that will carry you through the roughest times.

Discipline

When it comes to discipline, most faith-filled parents can be categorized in two ways: Those that spank and those that don't. Each of these parents, regardless of their view, feels passionate that they are in accordance with the Bible. But with such opposing positions, somebody must be wrong. Right?

Proverbs 13:24 He who spares the rod hates his son, but he who loves him is careful to discipline him.

Proverbs 19:18 Discipline your son, for in that there is hope; do not be a willing party to his death.

Proverbs 22:15 Folly is bound up in the heart of a child, but the rod of discipline will drive it far from him.

Proverbs 23:13-14 Do not withhold discipline from a child; if you punish him with the rod, he will not die. Punish him with the rod and save his soul from death.

Proverbs 29:15 The rod of correction imparts wisdom, but a child left to himself disgraces his mother.

Proverbs 29:17 Discipline your son, and he will give you peace; he will bring delight to your soul.

Discipline, without a doubt, is a natural part of parenting. We all need discipline, regardless of age, in order to be obedient believers. With it, we live. Without it, we die. Discipline is an unequivocal must.

But the debate isn't over *if* we should discipline. Instead, it lies in *how* we discipline, and the interpretation of the word *rod.*

Parents who are in favor of *gentle discipline*, or discipline without spanking, often argue that the word *rod* is used as a figure of speech. They feel that it merely represents discipline, and does not condone hitting a child.

On the other hand, some parents believe that the word *rod* is specifically pertaining to a physical rod used for hitting. They feel that this is the only effective disciplinary method.

After discussing this issue with many faith-filled parents, I've come to the conclusion that there may not be a clear-cut answer to the discipline dilemma. Different methods of discipline have proven to be very effective with different children. Maybe no single disciplinary measure is appropriate for all scenarios or personality types.

As a parent, your main goal should be to provide rules, guidance, and boundaries for your children of all ages. Just like us, children need the absolute values of the Bible. The Bible does not change, therefore supplying us with consistent instruction. Children need this same consistent instruction via consistent parenting. They need to know what is right, what is wrong, and the consequences, as well as the rewards, of their actions. When children know exactly what is expected of them, they are better equipped to act accordingly. They are also less reluctant to accept the punishment that awaits them if they disobey.

What I urge you *not* to do is to adopt the disciplinary

measures of your own parents for the simple sake of doing so. Instead, think it through and choose a method that works for your family. Meet your child with the level of punishment that fits the crime, and never over-discipline or discipline out of anger. Some actions do deserve more severe punishment, possibly a spanking. Other actions deserve less severe punishment, such as a time-out. But most types of disobedience can be resolved by a strong rebuke and gentle guidance.

In the end, it is your parental responsibility to discipline your children to the degree necessary for them to be obedient in the ways of the Lord. And, if you find that your children are in constant need of harsh discipline, the time has come for *you* to reevaluate your parenting technique.

Entertainment

Children are impressionable. They absorb everything that they come into contact with, whether good or bad. And in today's society, the television is in the spot light.

Many children spend hours upon hours watching programs–many of which are inappropriate for young eyes. Toddlers are often "baby-sat" by their favorite cartoon friend, picking up immoral behaviors and warped values.

Parents often underestimate the power of television. Besides any particular show's overall message, children are targeted by self-seeking advertisers. They are swamped with misinformation, and tempted by places, foods, and toys. This is all done in the name of money.

Too much television, over an hour a day for a toddler, has a negative impact on their mental capabilities for the rest of their lives. It is an inadvertent catalyst in the dumbing-down of America.

Parents must be strongly cautioned about what they choose to allow their children to watch. Many children's shows have inappropriate language, violence, and anti-God messages. They are often about passing gas, witchcraft, criticizing others, and unbiblical holidays. If we want our children to grow up to be God-abiding citizens, we must eliminate this moral filth. Children are impressionable–so let those impressions be Godly ones.

Schooling

Most faith-filled parents readily acknowledge that America's public school system is corrupt. Yet strangely, many of these parents still permit their children to attend. Maybe this is due to plain ignorance. Or maybe it revolves around procrastination, money, or inexcusable laziness. Either way, America's children are bearing the ultimate burden. They are encouraged to take the wide road that is full of sin, and are possibly forfeiting their eternal lives.

1 Corinthians 15:33 Do not be misled: "Bad company corrupts good character."

God commands that our children are to meditate on Him night and day–a lifestyle that cannot occur in the pagan school system. Instead, children are being taught the polluted ways of this world–to accept the unacceptable. And as Scripture warns, they are also being corrupted by their peers. Peer pressure is a very real thing, and no child is exempt.

A handful of believing parents claim to be doing the work of God by sending their children to public schools. Like arrows in the Lord's army, they expect their biblically-immature youth to resist evil and fight for the greater good.

Unfortunately, these parents are sadly mistaken. Children are just that–children. The word *child* means *a young human being below the age of full physical development*. Not only is a child physically immature, but spiritually as well. They are vulnerable and unequipped to resist the ever-increasing evil. Instead, they are being overtaken by evil, because an unprepared army sent to battle will fail.

Another concern that arises within the institution of public education is that it enables the secular government to brainwash youth in mass proportions. These easily-influenced children are being taught to accept new-age philosophies, such as "do what feels good to you." They are also encouraged to accept unbiblical practices.

For example, students are taught to be tolerant of homosexuality because it is *an acceptable means of sexual orientation*. They are also taught that people who oppose homosexuality are terrorists. Even the most biblically-inept individual knows the Lord's stance on unnatural sexual practices. This is just the beginning of Christianity being labeled as terroristic. Why should our children bear the brunt of these fallacies?

The Bible warns that this world is self-destructive, and we are gradually climbing toward the end times. With the one world currency already launched and the increasing talk of unity, the end is near. Children need the Word of God now more than ever. So why subject them to thirteen years of worldly views?

Proverbs 22:6 Train a child in the way he should go, and when he is old he will not turn from it.

This verse is vital to effective parenting. If you train a child in the way he should go, he will not turn from it! This is wonderful news for God-abiding parents–but it can backfire. If the school system is allowed to train your child, he will also not turn from it. So it is crucial for you to take charge and train your children in the ways of the Lord.

The word *train* means *to be taught a particular skill or type of behavior through regular practice and instruction*. Training a child on the weekends and evenings is *not* regular practice and instruction. Instead, it must be done on a daily basis–similar to what the public schools are doing.

Deuteronomy 11:18-20 Fix these words of mine in your hearts and minds; tie them as symbols on your hands and bind them on your foreheads. Teach them to your children, talking about them when you sit at home and when you walk along the road, when you lie down and when you get up. Write them on the doorframes of your houses and on your gates. . .

In order to successfully train your children, you must train them all of the time–sitting at home, walking along the road, always! It is impossible to do this unless your children are with you the majority of the time. Training your children is a full-time job–and your God-given duty as a faith-filled parent.

Christian school is another option, but a more expensive one. In addition, how would any parent know precisely what their child is being taught? With such major doctrinal differences among believers, children can easily be misinformed by an instructor's warped perception. For that very reason, it is vital for a parent to educate their own children.

2 Timothy 3:16-17 All Scripture is God-breathed and is useful for teaching, rebuking, correcting and training in righteousness, so that the man of God may be thoroughly equipped for every good work.

When it comes to home schooling, some parents are intimidated by their perceived lack of ability or qualification. However, the only thing a parent needs to be qualified is the Bible! The Lord has provided all parents with a manual to train their children, and themselves as well. It is a manual that cannot be altered or outdated. It is the Book of Life.

Home schooling is the most natural and God-honoring way a parent can educate their children. It also prevents the myriad of insecurities that children develop when forced to fend for themselves at the age of five. Home schooled children are nurtured in the safety of their own homes and are taught by the only people who love them unconditionally–their parents. These children are consistently taught God's ways and the necessary skills for real life. Home education is just another extension of parent/child bonding with immeasurable results.

Some parents worry that a home schooled child won't be socialized, but who has socialization helped? Even so, home schooled children are well-socialized, even where their public school peers are lacking. They are able to comfortably interact with adults, as well as other children. They also tend to be easy-going, respectful, and confident.

The cost of home schooling is very reasonable, all dependent on which method you plan to use. The least expensive route would be to create your own curriculum package. Simply decide what you want and need to teach, find the age-appropriate books, and make a schedule. The more expensive option is to buy prepared lesson plans. There are many companies that specifically sell home schooling curriculum for believers, and you can choose one that suits you and your child. From basic subjects such as reading, writing, and arithmetic, to extracurricular activities and languages, teach your child as you feel led. Use the Bible as your central guide.

Your child has been learning from you for the first five years of his or her life. Why can't it continue? There is nobody better equipped than you. Your child is your most precious commodity and most important responsibility. Embrace what the Lord has blessed you with, and home educate your child in His ways.

To Work or Not to Work?

In today's society, a working woman is not a rarity. Women have indeed proven themselves, and have successfully dispelled the myth that females are inferior. Many of these women juggle a demanding career as well as a family–but at what expense?

Being a wife and mother is a full-time job. Who can be thoroughly devoted to two full-time jobs? Nobody. One job will be neglected, and this is usually the role of wife and mother.

Problems arise when we neglect our God-given career for one that brings us money. Children of working mothers are often left alone, placed in a daycare, or sent to public school. Considering the negative impact all of these actions have on our youth, is it worth it? More than that, is this good stewardship and acceptable by the Lord?

When a child is placed in your womb, it isn't a haphazard act of nature. Instead, it is a part of the Lord's plan for your life. It is a responsibility given directly unto you–the mother.

If the Lord meant for someone else to care for or teach your child, your child would have been born to someone else. But he or she wasn't. He or she was born to you–the mother, the childcare provider, and the teacher. The Lord has called you to a purpose, and it is vital to fulfill your God-given career.

Joshua 1:8 Do not let this Book of the Law depart from your mouth; meditate on it day and night, so that you may be careful to do everything written in it. Then you will be prosperous and successful.

As a faith-filled mother, you're responsible for having your child meditate on God's Word day and night. This is a task of vital importance, and cannot be placed in the hands of another individual. You are personally responsible for your child's well-being, physically and spiritually. It is *your* job. And no where in the Bible does the Lord permit for you to pass off this responsibility to someone else–whether a public school teacher or daycare provider.

Just like public schools, daycares are clearly unfit for God's children. Children are vulnerable and susceptible to a myriad of worldly iniquities. Each year, thousands of cases of neglect, molestation, and abuse come from daycares. These cases occur in the most unsuspecting places, catching even the most observant person by surprise.

In addition, the overall environment in a daycare is institutional and children are treated in a very clinical manner. Newborn babies are left to cry themselves to sleep. Toddlers aren't allowed to receive the affection that they so deeply desire. Children are forced to adhere to rigid standards with scheduled lunch times, nap times, and play times. And illness spreads like wildfire through contaminated diapers, bottles, and sippie cups. Not to mention the cost–averaging one third to one half of an individual's weekly pay.

Instinctually, most mothers know that sending their children to daycare is wrong. Quite often, a mother sheds just as many tears as the child during the initial separation. This separation does become easier for both–the mother desensitizes herself, and the child is forced to deal with the harsh reality that mommy isn't coming back until later.

What the working mother needs to realize is that the Lord does not expect her to sacrifice her children for means of survival. Being a stay-at-home wife and mother is more valuable than any career–it is a God-given duty and not one to neglect. Plus, when we do things God's way, He will bless us abundantly.

Some mothers are faced with the unfortunate situation where they must work because the husband/father is not around. This is an exception and the mother needs to make the best of a bad situation. Maybe close friends or family members can lend a helping hand. Maybe the mother can earn a living by caring for other children in her home.

Other mothers are often interested in making a little extra income–which is fine, as long as the side-job is secondary. There are many money-making opportunities for stay-at-home mom's–ones that won't interfere with her ultimate responsibility–her family.

Chapter Six

The birth of our children is something that we remember for the rest of our lives. Whether good or bad, it leaves a lasting impression. It shapes us as women, and sets us on the path of motherhood. And it is vital that this experience be safe, satisfying, and dignified.

Unfortunately, many births do not always turn out as we have dreamed. It is then that we are left with anger, hurt, fear, resentment, and loneliness. Oftentimes, we search for the reason that things ended up as they did.

The following is a piece that I wrote about four years ago, after the birth of my first child. This birth was a horrific event that left me with many scars. It also left me with an unyielding desire to experience birth as the Lord intended—naturally.

The Lasting Pain of Childbirth

It has been a year now, almost two, since the most traumatic and life-altering event of my life—the birth of my daughter. Vivid images and intense sorrow have branded my memory. Flashbacks occur without warning. Most of all, I am haunted by the unbearable feeling of my body being violated.

I'm not sure what is more painful–the actual event, or that what was done to me was not only legal, but also routine. One thing that I am sure of is that time hasn't healed.

Finding out that I was pregnant was the most miraculous moment of my life. The entire world could have vanished that day, and my husband and I wouldn't have noticed. We were consumed by the incredible knowledge that we were going to be parents.

Common sense and intuition ruled out the possibility of a hospital birth. Although I briefly considered an unassisted home-birth, my husband wasn't comfortable with it. So we mutually agreed on a midwife-assisted birth in a freestanding birthing center. As first-time parents, this decision seemed wise.

My pregnancy passed by smoothly and without a single complication. I thoroughly enjoyed every moment, and optimism radiated from my very being. My faith, which was unwavering, left me filled with peace throughout the days and nights–nights that were spent marveling over the moment that I'd meet my precious baby.

Early one morning, around the forty-second week of my pregnancy, I awoke to a single gush of fluid. This gush continued on as a constant trickle, leaving no question as to whether I were in labor or not, for I certainly was. My waters had broken.

Immediately, adrenaline rushed throughout my body. I was no longer a mother-in-waiting, but a mother-in-labor. The time had finally come.

My husband called the birthing center, and I was sadly aware that my favorite midwife wasn't going to answer. She had suddenly relocated the prior week, uprooting my vision of the perfect birth.

Instead, my least-favorite midwife was on call. I hadn't bonded with her during the entire pregnancy because she was insensitive and impatient. The news of her presence was distressing, to say the least.

However, as disappointing as it may have been, the

unfortunate situation quickly vanished from my mind. Nothing could overshadow the thrill of knowing that my baby was about to be born.

I labored at home for about twelve hours. I walked, breathed, relaxed, and meticulously charted my progress. Although my contractions were unorganized, they were progressively becoming stronger. The time had come to test my endurance and I was ready for the challenge.

As the contractions strengthened, it didn't take long for my anxious husband to suggest going to the birthing center. I agreed. As a first-time-mother, I didn't know exactly what to expect. This way, we could bar any unexpected surprises.

Upon arrival, the midwife examined me. I was only two centimeters dilated. This news was disappointing, for I had expected to be further along.

Fortunately, the baby and I were in excellent health. Everything was progressing just as it should, and all I needed was a bit of rest. Because it was late, the midwife suggested that we remain there.

Early the next morning, my contractions had grown more intense, but they were easily bearable. I hadn't dilated much, so I spent hours walking around, trying to help the labor to progress.

As I labored peacefully, watching the heavy March snow fall on the city below, the midwife informed me that my time was running out. It had almost been twenty-four hours since my waters initially broke, and it was their policy to transfer a client to the hospital at that point.

During birth preparation classes, this scenario was briefly mentioned. It was also labeled as a rarity and of no concern. However, this "rarity" was now threatening my natural birth. A mere technicality had the authority to sentence me–a healthy woman with a healthy baby–to a hospitalized labor and delivery. What was I to do?

Twenty-four hours came and went, and I made every attempt

to help the labor along. The tension was rising, to say the least. I was fearful–no, terrified–of what lay ahead, and the recollection of hospital birth horror stories flashed through my mind. Was I going to be the next victim?

The midwife did one final exam and I nervously awaited the results. Every fiber of my being hoped and prayed that I had somehow made rapid progress. If so, maybe she'd let me continue on. Maybe my dreams wouldn't be completely shattered. Maybe I'd be given a chance to allow nature to take it's course–a course that was well under way, even if a bit more sluggish than one would had hoped for.

The midwife looked up at me with a grim expression on her face. I was only four centimeters dilated. Although the baby and I were in excellent health, she decided to transfer us to the hospital. It was a terrifying realization, but even my worse fears didn't lead me to anticipate the horrific events that were about to unfold.

Without delay, I gathered my belongings, leaving behind the video camera that I had pre-positioned to record the miraculous event. Fear swept over me like a raging storm, and panic jolted my inmost being. I was frail, confused, and in the midst of an ever-increasing battle with the forces brewing within.

Considering the vulnerability of my predicament, I desperately needed someone to rely on. So trusting that the midwife had my best interests at heart, I didn't even resist the transfer. It was a terrible decision, although I didn't know it at the time. It was a decision that would bring me a lifetime of regret.

As expected, the hospital was bright and un-welcoming, causing my entire body to become rigid with fear. As a result, my contractions suddenly worsened, making my manageable labor anything but manageable. I moaned in severe pain.

Despite my anguish, I stubbornly refused the wheelchair that was promptly brought to my aid. I just couldn't submit that easily, although the odds were now against me. Instead, I stumbled down the long corridor, as independently as I could, to the bleak destiny that awaited.

Immediately upon entering the stiff and sterile room, I was abruptly told to change into an old, lifeless gown. I did, my identity was erased, and I had officially become hospital property.

Following in the footsteps of the women before, the outcome wasn't promising. I was heading full-force in the wrong direction, being too distraught and preoccupied to retaliate.

I was then told to lie on a narrow hospital bed. A doctor swiftly entered the room, briefly introduced herself, and took the liberty of spreading my legs apart. I was still only four centimeters dilated.

Disappointment glared in her eyes as she shook her head, peeled off the rubber glove, and disappeared into the crowd of medical personnel.

Following the exam, I was not allowed up from the hospital bed. A fetal monitor was strapped around my pregnant belly and a blood pressure cuff was attached to my arm. I was immobile.

With no chance to work with the intensifying pangs that wreaked havoc on my body, I lay in agony. My laboring moans quickly annoyed the irritable hospital staff, who put no effort in hiding their feelings. I was showered with displeasing glares and the stern warning that if I wanted to continue on, I had to have pain medication.

My frightened husband stood next to me, speechless. My midwife, who was supposedly present to voice my concerns, stood uselessly in the corner. I felt abandoned, and my bedridden state gave the labor pains full reign, leaving me weeping and wailing.

After succumbing to an epidural, I was paralyzed from the waste down. Repeatedly, my body was intimately violated. My private parts were openly exposed and tampered with, leaving me feeling sexually humiliated and degraded. But it wasn't over.

The doctor wasn't satisfied with how the fetal monitor was functioning, so she opted for an internal fetal monitor. Without my consent, she parted my legs and screwed the metal spring-like device into my unborn baby's head. I could feel the wire hanging out of me.

At that point, my mind was already whirling with a storm of emotions. My opinion and privacy had absolutely no value, and I was deliberately made to feel inadequate and uneducated. Even worse, my helpless baby was now being assaulted and victimized within my womb. How could someone do that to an unborn child?

The impatient doctor was frustrated with how slowly I was dilating. Although my baby and I were not medically distressed, she decided to induce my labor with the all-too-common drug Pitocin. It was administered through an I.V. and caused my perfectly healthy baby to go into fetal distress.

The doctor tampered with the Pitocin for quite a while. When my baby became distressed, she would discontinue the drug. My baby would then stabilize. Once the drug was restarted, my baby would again become distressed. The doctor's unnecessary intervention was clearly causing complications, but she wouldn't stop.

Numerous people were entering and leaving the room. The atmosphere was unfriendly, impersonal, and down right hectic. Yet despite the spectators, the doctor openly examined me. She then selfishly decided that she wouldn't allow my labor to progress. In the interest of saving time, she preferred a Cesarean section.

The word 'Cesarean' echoed within my scattered mind, but I was so drugged and in shock that everything seemed unreal. I tried desperately to wake up because I knew that it must have been a nightmare. And it was, but I was wide awake.

From the moment I had entered the hospital, reality became a blur. Whether due to fear, stress, vulnerability, the liberal use of drugs, or the condescending hospital personnel, I gradually felt as though I had been drowning. I sank deeper and deeper as the delivery deviated from my expectations of a natural birth. My mind raced haphazardly, and I was unable to fully grasp what was happening, let alone defend myself. What was happening? Why me? Where did I go wrong? Why was no one standing up for me? With utter despair, I watched. I waited.

Then suddenly, like a welcoming lifeboat, I felt the unmistakable urge to push. Excited and hopeful, I announced it to the entire room. But I was wrongfully ignored. I pleaded for someone to listen, but my plea fell on deaf ears. My only hope vanished and the world buzzed on around me.

Modesty was obviously not a consideration as I was shaved in preparation for the surgery. I was then told to move my numb, pregnant body from one narrow hospital bed to another. Vulnerable, like a beached whale, I was at the mercy of all who decided to poke and prod.

I was wheeled off to a bright, metallic operating room. To add to my susceptibility, my quivering arms were pulled away from my body and tied down. Simultaneously, a drape was hung in front of my face. Not only did it hide from me what the doctor was doing, but from her view, it depersonalized me. She could now heartlessly view me as a specimen, not a human.

Bound like a criminal, I was drugged, nauseated, and shaking uncontrollably. Despite the epidural, I could feel the scalpel slicing through the layers of my pregnant flesh. A wet suction noise droned from behind the drape, and I felt cold, dreadfully ill, and terrified.

In a twisted, yet somehow medically-legal way, I had been raped. And now I was going to be robbed of the birth of my baby. There was nothing that I could do—nothing that anybody could do. In the battle of good versus evil, evil had a victory.

With a swoop of immense, uncomfortable pressure, my innocent baby was violently ripped from the safety of my womb. There was no crying and no momentous first glance. My eyes only saw a naked, lifeless body swiftly pass by in the gloved hands of a stranger.

At that very moment, something much more than the umbilical cord had been severed. A bond had been building between my baby and I during the previous nine months. But that single moment that would have solidified that bond–the moment we'd meet face to face–was taken away.

The doctor patted herself on the back and received praise from her on looking colleagues. She had another Cesarean under her belt and the delusion that she had saved yet another baby.

I awoke sometime later in a small, dimly lit room. I was alone, incredibly thirsty, and unable to move. I felt so awful that my only thought was of how desperately I wanted to die.

I then awoke in a larger room–a room with sunlight peering through shaded windows. It was the following day, and my husband was there with our newborn daughter. He was smiling, as proud as could be, and handed me this tiny, tightly wrapped bundle.

That moment was the first time that I held my baby . . . I think. Tears filled my adoring eyes, but she didn't feel like mine. Along with me, I felt that my baby had died.

A nurse entered the room and vividly reminded me of the incomprehensible humiliation. She checked my incision and happily commented on what a beautiful job the doctor had done. She then proceeded to remove my catheter and change my bloodied pads. There I was, a grown woman, with a stranger changing my bloodied pads in broad daylight. I was too ashamed to even look at my husband.

The remainder of my hospital stay proved to be an incessant battle. I even had to defend my right to breast-feed. I was continually encouraged to give my baby formula, and I sternly refused. This angered the nurses, but breast-feeding was too important to compromise.

My husband and I guarded against vaccinations, the eye ointment, and the vitamin K injection. For our baby's protection, we didn't allow her out of our sight. Enough damage had been done, and we had to prevent her from being subjected to further trauma.

I returned home a day or so later. Breast-feeding seemed

impossible, but I wouldn't give up. It was the only thing I had left. It was the only thing that the hospital didn't take from me, despite how hard they tried.

Soon after, postpartum depression took over. I didn't adjust well to being a mother, and I felt completely detached from my baby. Most of all, I couldn't bear what the hospital had done to me.

Day and night I would cry uncontrollably. No matter how much I cried, I couldn't release the relentless pain that I was feeling. I was inconsolable. I couldn't eat, get out of bed, or even begin to rationalize my feelings.

Days and weeks passed. I came to a point where I would cry, yet no more tears would emerge. I truly felt beyond healing. I didn't care about myself, my husband, or my new baby who needed me. I lost all faith.

My loving husband, who somehow managed to care for a helpless newborn and a helpless wife, tried desperately to find a solution. The birthing center proved to be useless. Apparently, but not surprisingly, postpartum depression only occurs in women who deliver in a hospital. Every doctor we consulted refused to help me because I wouldn't take medication. It was hopeless.

After a few weeks, the depression eased up. I contribute it to my husband's willingness to encourage and care for me, and the unfailing power of prayer. I was finally able to perform minimal duties, and most important, interact with my baby. Although I still didn't feel quite like myself, I was heading in a positive direction. I was regaining control of my life–of a life that still seemed beyond repair.

I awoke one night during a hospital nightmare–something that had plagued me often. My heart was racing. My skin was burning. Immense and relentless pressure squeezed my lungs, while overwhelming fear and panic swept over my body. It was my first panic attack.

Stumbling over to the adjoining bathroom, I removed my shirt and bra in a desperate attempt to relieve the pressure. I did anything imaginable to escape the breath-robbing compression of my lungs, even causing myself to vomit. Then suddenly, while rolling on the bathroom floor in a frenzy, the symptoms all together ceased.

The same thing occurred a week or so later. This time, it was much stronger and lasted much longer. Horrified, I truly thought that I was going to go crazy. The pain and pressure were debilitating. My mind raced haphazardly, and every attempt to gain control failed. So my husband called an ambulance.

The unprofessional paramedics didn't take me to the emergency room, which they were later reprimanded for. Instead, they took me to the maternity ward, assuming that I was having a postpartum-related issue.

The doctor wanted to examine my uterus, which I explained was unnecessary. I felt confident that I was having a panic attack, and more distress would only make matters worse.

As expected, she ignored me. She was the almighty doctor and I was merely a clueless patient. So out of intimidation, I submitted to her request. My pride was again diminished and my body was intimately violated. This wasted time and humiliation only proved that I was fine.

My husband and daughter arrived shortly after, and I was transported to the appropriate section of the hospital.

After waiting for hours, my attack long gone, I finally saw a doctor. She monitored my heart, took x-rays, and concluded what I already knew. I was having panic attacks. I was given a prescription, which I never filled, and went home.

I spent the next few weeks having one attack after another. My only relief from the anxiety was when I was asleep. I slept when the baby slept. We lived in bed.

During that time, I never considered taking medication. Compromising my baby's health for my comfort was not an option. Instead, I needed the true healing that came from the Lord above.

So one day I woke up and decided that I refused to live this way. The person that I had become was unknown to me. The real me was strong and independent, yet I had become frail and afraid.

So I forced myself out of bed and struggled through the extreme anxiety in order to perform daily chores. It was the most difficult thing that I had ever done, but each day became easier than the previous. It was my turning point.

Since then, I have spent much of my mother/daughter time trying to compensate for the violent way that she entered the world. I also try to make up for lost time. Although we had a rough start, I am positive that she and I are as close as humanly possible. Not only do I contribute it to nursing, but largely to co-sleeping and being a stay-at-home mom. We are always together, just like a mother and child should.

The hospital contributes my Cesarean to the umbilical cord being wrapped around my daughter's neck. Babies are often born with wrapped cords and it is never a cause for a Cesarean. The doctor simply needed to create an excuse for her harsh, extreme, and inhumane behavior.

I am deeply saddened that between my husband and my midwife, nobody helped my daughter or me. But I have now realized that my husband was also a victim. He was silenced and intimidated by the hospital's false confidence and sense of urgency.

The physical scar from the incision has healed, although it visually serves as a daily reminder. It signifies the unjust, horrible way my dear daughter entered the world. My heart is filled with sorrow as I recall how brutally we had both been treated. My daughter was denied a natural, gentle passage into this world. As for me, a doctor fondled with my innermost self–parts that not even I have seen or touched.

The only thing I've gained from this experience is a justified distrust toward the entire medical establishment. They surpassed my worst expectations and solidified my intuitive assumptions. They unveiled how warped modern medicine really is–a barbaric profession clothed in technology.

Something was taken from me on that snowy March day. I lost more than my pride and my dignity. I lost myself.

Since then, I have still been trying to make up for lost time with my daughter. I am saddened that her birth story isn't a pleasant one, but I try to emphasize the positive aspects. I remember the joy of discovering that the Lord had healed me of infertility. I reminisce of the nine months of a purely wonderful pregnancy. It wasn't all bad.

I seldom talk about my daughter's birth around her because I don't want her to feel bad. When I look at her, I don't recall the pain and sorrow of her birth. Instead, I feel a bond with her because we experienced it together. More than anything, I feel guilt because I should have protected her. I had three choices: To rely on a doctor; to rely on a midwife, or to rely on God. I know better now.

This is not to say that all midwife-assisted births turn out this way. Many women have beautiful, safe, and satisfying births with certified and lay midwives. You just need to weigh the risks.

During that time in my life, I can honestly say that I lost all faith. I didn't understand how the Lord could let that happen to me. I felt that I had been faithful, and yet all the faith in the world couldn't save me. But my thoughts have changed.

I now realized that we don't always understand why things happen, and we just need to accept that they did. I feel that I have learned a lot from that experience. I also feel that I can help other women deal with their hurtful birth experiences.

After that birth, I knew that there must be a better way. I spent the first year of my daughter's life researching alternatives. It was an obsession, really. But I needed to find the answer. And as you'll see in the following chapter, I did.

Traumatic Birth

When an envisioned birth turns out to be anything but

dreamlike, many mothers are left with mere disappointment. Yet some births stray much further from the expectant mother's dreams. And depending upon her perception and reaction of the events that took place, she may be mildly affected or completely shattered–even to the point of taking her own life.

When it comes to a birth-gone-wrong, modern obstetrics is usually the culprit. From high-tech gadgets, to false threats, to authoritative and condescending medical personnel, the overall atmosphere is one of fear and forced submission. Birth is turned into a Broadway show with the mother's genitals in the spotlight, leaving no question as to why so many women fall into a downward spiral.

After a traumatic birth, most women will experience a myriad of mixed emotions. These emotions are often misunderstood, resulting in thoughtless comments from well-meaning friends and family members. They may tell the mother that she should be happy that her baby turned out okay. She may be told that she is overreacting or being ungrateful. Or she may be told to just get over it. But it isn't that easy.

Just like other victims, the victims of modern obstetrics deserve the right to be angry, sad, disappointed, frustrated, and regretful. They need time to heal. Although what happened may have been legal, it was wrong. And as a midwife once put it, it is "medicalized rape."

Dealing with the feelings associated with rape is a difficult task on its own. However, the victim of modern obstetrics has a double-blow. Not only does she have to deal with being legally raped, but also the terror of having the life of her unborn baby threatened.

Oftentimes, trust and abandonment issues develop after a traumatic birth. The mother had entrusted her very life with her abuser–the doctor, while close friends and family members witnessed the horrific event without intervening. That kind of abuse and abandonment is life-shattering and difficult for anyone to fathom.

Depending on the woman and the nature of her labor and delivery, she may experience *postpartum depression* or *post-traumatic stress disorder*, among other things. These disorders are serious, and should not be mistaken for the temporary emotional upset known as the *baby blues*.

The baby blues is something that many women experience within the first week or so after the birth. It may go unnoticed, but is generally characterized by random crying spells and a sudden, *but momentary*, shift from happiness to sadness. The cause is usually hormonal and will balance out on its own.

Postpartum depression, on the other hand, is much more serious. It can begin immediately after the birth, or anywhere within the first year. Sometimes the onset is even later. Postpartum depression, also known as PPD, is characterized by appetite and sleep changes, crying, irritability, and a sense of hopelessness. In extreme cases, it may even cause suicidal thoughts, requiring immediate medical attention.

Along with postpartum depression, post-traumatic stress disorder is another likely problem after a traumatic birth. It is characterized by panic attacks, nightmares about the traumatic event, and flashbacks.

If you are experiencing any of these disorders, know that the Lord can pull you through. No matter how unreachable you may feel, He can do it. Not doctors. Not drugs. Healing comes from the Lord, and in trusting Him wholeheartedly. Also know that you are not alone. Thousands of women experience disappointing and traumatic births each year. Maybe one day our voices will be heard.

Vaginal Birth After Cesarean

Cesarean deliveries are commonplace in today's hospitals, many of which are performed for no other reason than mere preference. Once a woman has undergone this surgical delivery, she is forever labeled as *high risk*. And she is high risk *if* she delivers in a hospital.

A hospital, which is an institution dedicated to the ill, is a dangerous place for all expecting women. Healthy women are viewed as being plagued by a serious disease–pregnancy, while Cesarean victims are seen as ticking time-bombs on the verge of exploding.

Having a past Cesarean immediately triggers the use of *any* and *every* means of intervention–including a repeat Cesarean. This is done out of the perceived threat of *uterine rupture,* an unlikely condition unless doctor-induced.

As past and present studies prove, having a vaginal birth is always safer, whether a woman has had a previous Cesarean or not. Even so, most doctors tend to adhere to their preset beliefs, regardless of how outdated and irrational they may be. These doctors may allow a "trial" labor, with their high-tech equipment and extreme interventions posing further complications.

Among these interventions may be the induction of labor–a procedure that is dangerous for the Cesarean and non-Cesarean mother alike. Induction drugs cause unnatural and extreme contractions–contractions that can rupture even an intact uterus. Considering that it is uterine rupture which supposedly makes a Cesarean mother high risk, why increase her chances with such a contradictory procedure?

The term *uterine rupture* immediately brings about the vivid image of a uterus bursting open, spilling out its contents, and hemorrhaging uncontrollably. However, this simply isn't the case.

Instead, the uterus merely splits at the incision site when it can't withstand the rigors of labor. This can occur in *any* woman, whether she has had a Cesarean delivery or not. If this scenario does occur, the Cesarean mother is actually better off. Her incision will have a clean separation which is easier to repair, unlike the intact uterus which would rupture haphazardly.

Certain factors do make a woman more at risk for uterine

rupture. The most prominent is the type of incision she has. There are three types: Classical, which is a high, vertical incision; low transverse, which is a low, horizontal incision; and low vertical, which is self-explanatory.

The low transverse incision is the most common one, and the safest. It has the most integrity of all the incisions and rarely splits open. Please note, however, that the uterine incision is *different* from the abdominal incision. Although often the same, the visible abdominal incision may not be in the same direction or location as the uterine incision.

When planning to birth at home, it is important for a Cesarean mother to know, as a precaution, the signs of uterine rupture. The main signs are a boardlike uterus that will not contract, abdominal pain, abdominal swelling, bleeding, a rise in pulse and a drop in blood pressure, and fever. Unfortunately, some of these symptoms can indicate anything or nothing at all.

One important thing to note is that many Cesarean victims do feel abdominal pain or tenderness in late pregnancy and during labor. In most cases, this discomfort is benign and does not indicate uterine rupture. If more specific signs are present, then there may be a cause for concern and further measures should be taken to ensure the safety of the mother and her unborn child.

If you are a Cesarean victim, know that it is *not* a contradiction to having a midwife-assisted birth or a home-birth. It is important to be informed and aware, and crucial to be spiritually prepared. Many times, Cesarean victims are left feeling incapable of delivering a baby vaginally, let alone naturally without intervention. This is an ideal foothold for the devil. But you are capable!

The Lord has created your body to have babies, and He can heal even the deepest of scars. Build your faith and choose to fully rely on Him. Let go of your fear, let go of your concern, and let the Lord lead you to where He wants you to go. He will meet you at your level of faith. He wants what is best for you and your baby, and His way–the natural way, is the best.

Chapter Seven

It is human nature for different people to handle things in different ways. As for me, I am a writer. Whenever I experience intense emotions of any kind, I immediately look for a pencil and a piece of paper. It is a pull within that I can't resist, and a way to express myself, even when no one else is interested.

After the birth of my second child, I was just as eager to write as I was after the birth of my first. This time, however, I was bubbling over with positive and joyous emotions. So I wrote, and then I wrote some more. Let me take you on the journey of my healing home-birth.

A Healing Home-Birth

Despite my efforts, the birth of my first child went horribly wrong. My natural, midwife-assisted birth turned into an unnatural, doctor-assisted Cesarean. To make matters worse, it was unnecessary.

Once I returned home, the trauma didn't cease. As the drugs wore off and I reentered reality, I was consumed by the actualization of what had happened. I was left feeling sexually violated and humiliated, and needlessly cheated out of the birth of my daughter.

That was a rough first year. I was filled with sadness, resentment, and frustration. The simple thought of what had happened to me was unbearable. The mere mention of the words 'doctor' or 'hospital' would make me sick to my stomach and furious.

Shortly after my daughter's first birthday, I became pregnant with my second child. This time, delivering at the birthing center was not an option. As a Cesarean victim, I had earned the title of being 'high risk.' But this didn't concern me. Months of careful research had determined the path that I would travel. I was going to have an unassisted home-birth. It was the only way to ensure a safe birth for my baby and I.

I began my journey by taking an honest look at the basics of prenatal care. This included good nutrition, rest, exercise, and monitoring the baby. I was fully capable of performing all of these duties, as most women are, and nobody knew my body better than I did. So I logically concluded that I would perform my own prenatal care. Hiring a professional would not only be unnecessary, but foolish, considering that I am a non-interventionist.

First, I closely monitored my diet and ate mostly organic foods (opposed to only the easily accessible ones). I avoided colorings, preservatives, hormones, caffeine, and other toxins. I also continued to take a high-quality prenatal vitamin.

Next, I monitored my weight and blood pressure, and charted the progress periodically. I gained weight slowly in the beginning, as I had expected, and more rapidly later on. As for my blood pressure, it lingered on the higher end, but was stable and well-within normal limits. I made a mental note to keep an eye on it, and it never amounted to anything.

At twenty-eight weeks, I began to monitor the baby's movements–a simple way to assess his or her overall condition. I learned the baby's activity patterns and knew what to expect. If a drastic shift were to occur, further measures could be taken. Fortunately, that never happened.

My one-year-old made rest hard to come by, but the exercise was plentiful. I managed to nap when she would nap, and I enjoyed swimming in the summer months.

Throughout the pregnancy, I paid close attention to my body. I was aware of the signs and symptoms that could indicate a problem. I also spent a great deal of time researching the birthing process. Due to the interest I had previously, I was already quite knowledgeable. However, in order to feel confident about delivering my own baby, I needed to know more.

The Internet proved to be a valuable resource. It clearly discredited the popular notion that childbirth is volatile and dangerous. Most important, it reassured me that my body was capable of delivering a baby by itself, without intervention. As a woman, the Lord had created me completely equipped. Expecting complications was not only doubting His divine work, but also unfounded. Childbirth is involuntary and uncomplicated. It is just as safe as any other bodily function. But that didn't mean that I'd go about it completely unprepared.

Although an emergency was highly unlikely, my husband and I made ourselves aware of what could happen. We also knew what we could and couldn't handle. For instance, we knew that eating a portion of the placenta would stop hemorrhaging. Although this wasn't a pleasant thought, desperate times do call for desperate measures. We also learned techniques for delivering a breech baby, a baby with the cord wrapped around its neck, and infant resuscitation. Above all, we were aware of the situations that warrant emergency medical assistance.

I spent much of the pregnancy collecting various items for the delivery. Some items were necessary, such as sterilized white shoelaces and small pruning sheers to tie and cut the cord. Other items were precautionary, such as tinctures of Shepard's Purse to stop hemorrhaging, and Angelica to encourage the expulsion of a retained placenta. And other items, such as old towels and clean sheets, were within arms reach for convenience. I kept these items together and readily available for the delivery.

Strengthening my faith was a crucial factor in being able to fully rely on the body that the Lord had given me. I remained prayerful throughout the days and nights, especially when fear would creep up. I'd research my Bible for anything pertaining to childbirth, prayer, and faith. I'd write these things in my pregnancy planner and meditate on them daily.

Each night I would read my Bible aloud to myself, to my husband, and to my daughter. I practically clothed myself in the Word of God and built my faith so that I could stand on it effortlessly. I knew that I could have faith or fear. I chose to have faith. And I knew that faith would give me the birth that I had always dreamed of.

My husband and I didn't tell many people about our plans. We didn't need or want any negative criticism. Many people thought that delivering at a birthing center with a midwife was outrageous, dangerous, and unthinkable. We could only imagine how they would feel about this. For the most part, it was a wonderful secret that the two of us shared.

My pregnancy was enjoyable and uneventful (by medical standards). There were no needles, no uncomfortable, internal exams, and no inaccurate, worrisome tests. My days were filled with contentment and the anticipation of the forthcoming birth.

Each day I'd admire my ripening belly and sing to the little baby blooming within. It was, after all, the miracle of life. Not a week passed by where I didn't write to him or her in my baby journal. And not a moment escaped without thanking the Lord. I was filled with joy during every waking moment, and full of peace while I slept.

The joy that I felt seemed to baffle others. I had the pregnancy glow, even while hunched over the toilet bowl. But it wasn't because I experienced pregnancy differently than most. Instead, I perceived it differently. I saw it as the blessing that it truly was.

Toward the end of my pregnancy I felt confident and ready. All of the preparations had been made, and the only thing left to do was wait.

By the end of my fortieth week, I was still pregnant. Although I occasionally felt Braxton-Hicks contractions, they never progressed.

Forty-two weeks came and went, and I was still pregnant. On the verge of being overdue, I had encountered a crossroads in my journey. Would I intervene, or let nature take its course?

I knew what a doctor or midwife would do. They'd induce my labor in fear of a stillbirth. I could help the labor along myself, if I wanted to. But I needed to remember that I was under the care of God, not man. I could submit to Him, or to flawed human understanding. So I chose Him, and my faith and perseverance paid off.

The following day I awoke from a blissful afternoon nap with contractions. They were mild and continued throughout the evening.

Early the next morning, the contractions had become strong enough to disturb my sleep. I was unsure if I was experiencing true labor, but I was excited and eager.

By daybreak, my hunch was confirmed. The contractions had increased in intensity and were becoming predictable. Labor had definitely arrived, and I actively worked with my body's efforts. I walked from room to room, up the stairs and down the stairs. I squatted with each twinge, and continually changed position, knowing that these constant actions would help the labor to progress.

Midmorning brought about a new wave of labor pains. They were short, with a reasonable break in between, but extremely uncomfortable. Although quite a nuisance, the severity didn't compare to the ones that followed.

By noon, the contractions had grown horribly severe. They were unyielding–one right after another, only seconds apart, and lasting a minute each. I spent hours doing whatever I needed to do to manage the pain. I walked. I squatted. I took shower after shower. I grunted and shouted.

During this time, the toilet, of all places, proved to be the most comfortable. I sat forward on it, then backward. It didn't necessarily ease the pain, but helped to mentally open a passage for the baby to descend.   I could also frequently relieve myself, allowing even more room for the baby. So I propped a pillow on the clammy tank and rested my weary head.

Labor was turning out slightly different from what I had expected. Not only was it excruciating, but relaxation didn't make a difference. I could feel every spasm in my abdomen as well as my lower back. My back would cramp fiercely, causing me to arch it. It may have been due to awkward fetal positioning, but I didn't care. Exhausted, I longed for just one second to rest.

To add to my discomfort, I began feeling chills and nauseated. After vomiting once or twice, I assumed that I was in transition. But I wasn't sure. I was in too much pain to analyze anything.

By early evening, the contractions had become agonizing and intolerable. I willfully fought the emerging feelings of doubt and inadequacy. Although this was a classic sign that the birth was imminent, I didn't care. What if I was wrong? What if this was only the beginning? What if the pain worsened and became too much for me to bear?

I prayed to the Lord, and my doubtful feelings were replaced by ones of hope and encouragement. This drastic shift of emotion was caused by a small glob of blood-tinged mucus discharge. I had lost my mucus plug. I had gained progress.

I took another shower in a desperate attempt to ease the relentless pain. As I sat on the shower floor, allowing the steamy water to pound on my throbbing back, I questioned if it was humanly possible to endure this much suffering. I also felt more forgiving of the women who took pain medication.

About fifteen minutes later, I noticed a puddle of meconium-stained water beneath me. I wasn't alarmed, but thankful. My waters had broken, the end was in sight, and I felt encouraged to go on.

Shortly after, I sensed that something had changed. My contractions were still intense and painful, but not as sharp. In a way, I was blanketed by a subtle tranquility. It was strange, like the calm before the storm. Was this it?

Then suddenly, I felt this incredible urge to push. The sensation was overwhelming and uncontrollable. I felt like I needed to pass an enormous bowel movement, and I didn't care that I was in the shower. I pushed without any hesitation.

The sensation strengthened and my body became engrossed by an inexpressible force. My mind was swept away into another dimension of labor. And as I realized that the birth was near, anticipation bubbled throughout my weakening limbs.

I called to my husband in the adjoining bedroom and told him to prepare the bed. I then loosely wrapped myself in a towel and stumbled over to him.

The contractions were vigorous—one after another—leaving little time to even breathe. My body was consumed by pain and involuntary motions, making it difficult to assume any other position than semi-sitting. So I lay there, with my upper body resting on my arms, and braced myself for the delivery.

My daughter, who had been curiously observing the entire labor, climbed up next to me. She twisted my hair around her little fingers, put her other fingers in her mouth, and somehow managed to drift off to sleep. My labor must have been tiring for the both of us, and she quickly contented herself with her usual nap time routine.

As for my husband, he sat at the foot of the bed, as casual as could be, skimming through a childbirth book for last minute pointers. For him, the boring day was about to become much more interesting. The time had come to push, and as the baby catcher, he had a front row seat.

My entire body continued to be entranced by this inexpressible impulse to bear down. I actually found a mysterious pleasure in cooperating with my body's natural tendencies. It said push, and I pushed.

This stage of labor was like a roller coaster. I could feel the sensation building and building. I'd shout to release the escalating energy because it seemed more than I could contain. I'd braced myself for what was coming. Then the sensation would peak, and I'd push. I'd push and push, grunting and shouting all the while in a steady roar.

Then, unexpectedly, my husband could see the head. I was thrilled to discover that my brief efforts were so productive. I had expected a lengthy pushing stage since I had never delivered a baby vaginally, but the journey was almost over.

With a mirror in place, I pushed, and the head became visible. A sliver of dark, wet hair appeared, and I was filled with awe and encouragement as I saw my baby for the first time.

As I retracted my muscles, the head would disappear. Like a game of hide-and-go-seek, the baby would come and go with each crescendo. But it was only a matter of time until he or she would be here to stay.

All along, I knew that there was a baby inside of me. I watched it grow. I felt it kick. I planned its birth. Yet the moment I saw it–just a peek, I knew that this moment was real. I had dreamt of this for two years, and now my maternal longings were finally being fulfilled.

My husband touched the top of our unborn baby's head, and I did too. He expected it to be hard like a skull, but it wasn't. It was soft.

I pushed again, the baby crowned, and I resisted by closing my legs. It burned and felt too large to pass through my body. However, I knew that this resistance was God's natural way of preventing tears.

With the next contraction, I gave one vigorous push and the head was delivered. There it was, this full head of hair between my quivering legs. I couldn't believe it. I asked my husband if it was okay, but he didn't know.

During the next contraction, I held my breath and pushed two more times. With a forceful gush of blood and fluid, the baby's body swiftly entered the world. It was 5:00 p.m. The baby was silent and gray.

My husband quickly wiped the baby's face and it began to cry. It was a beautiful, alleviating sound. It was a sound that every woman awaits. It was the sound of birth. It was a sound that tugged on the depths of my soul, triggering an instantaneous flood of tears and emotions. And it was a sound that proved that I did it.

He placed the precious newborn on my bare belly, skin to skin, and covered us in an old towel. It was beautiful, empowering, miraculous, and most of all, healing. I had spent two years mourning the loss of something that I had never experienced, but now I had.

I asked my husband if it was a girl or boy, but he didn't know. Amid the exhilaration, the baby's sex was overlooked. So he lifted the towel and announced that it was a girl. We had another beautiful girl!

I put my daughter, Cheyenne Olivia, to my breast and she immediately latched on. There we were, in a puddle of cold, bodily fluids, still attached by the umbilical cord. It was a raw, natural moment.

After she nursed for over a half of an hour, my husband tied and cut the cord. He then weighed, measured, and dressed her. She weighed 9 pounds and was 20 inches long. I found satisfaction in knowing that I had delivered such a large baby without rupturing my sutured uterus.

An hour and a half later, the placenta had not been delivered, putting a slight damper on the joyous evening. My husband massaged my uterus to help it along, but it didn't seem to work. I then took a dropper-full of Angelica and I nursed the baby again.

All of a sudden, I felt my uterus beginning to contract. With barely enough time to hand my husband the baby, one push delivered the placenta. This immediately eased the growing tension.

We put the placenta in a bowl, checked it over, and it was complete. This marked the end of an extraordinary and successful delivery. We had experienced the miracle of life first hand, without intervention.

Later that evening, my husband and I ordered out dinner and two slices of cheesecake. Not only was this our newborn daughter's birthday, but it happened to be our older daughter's birthday too. We didn't plan it that way, but the Lord always has a way with numbers.

We put two candles in one slice of cheesecake for our oldest, Natalia Renee, and none in the other slice for our newest addition, Cheyenne Olivia. We then sang the birthday song to both of our precious daughters.

The delivery surpassed my highest expectations and my deepest longings. I was swept up into a whirlwind of uncontainable joy and ecstasy. I was bursting with happiness and eager to tell everyone about my profound experience. Most of all, I was thankful to the Lord. His miraculous works left me feeling renewed and whole. I had redeemed my womanhood.

Although nothing can replace what the hospital has so violently taken from me, my yearning for a natural birth has been fulfilled. In this alone, I've found healing.

Still to this day, and probably for the rest of time, my husband and I joyfully reminisce about our unassisted home-birth.

I often refer to it as our God-assisted home-birth. The Lord was with us on that day, and we witnessed the flawlessness of His work. All things are possible with Him.

In hindsight, I now realize why the relaxation techniques didn't make a difference in the midst of labor. It is because I didn't practice them beforehand. If I had, I am positive that I could have managed my pain better. Labor isn't the time to try new things that require concentration. Instead, advanced preparation is the key.

After discussing the birth with my husband, I also realized that my speculation during labor was correct. My extreme back pain was probably due to awkward fetal positioning, for my baby emerged face-up. Most babies emerge face-down, and then rotate to a face-up position as the shoulders are born.

If you are considering an unassisted home-birth, please think it through. Knowing the joy of a home-birth, I could never discourage anybody from experiencing it. But you do need to rely on faith. It is by faith that I endured the pain. It is by faith that I didn't become panicked. And it is by faith that everything worked out just as it should.

Overcoming Home-Birth Obstacles

There are many factors that may lead a doctor or midwife to label a woman as high risk. Whether the risk is real or not, is all dependent on the specific situation. Either way, this biased classification usually results in a woman choosing, by default, to take a medical approach to her pregnancy, labor, and delivery. Aggressive obstetric care may prove to be more dangerous than the woman's preexisting condition left alone.

The good news is, that in God, no woman is high risk. God can do anything, no matter how big or how small. There isn't a single thing that He can't handle. There isn't a single thing that He can't change. And there isn't a single thing that He won't do for those He loves.

A high-risk woman, regardless of what she may have been told, does have options. She must diligently research her condition and know what complications could arise. She must also look for ways to prevent or reverse what makes her high risk in the first place. Most important, she must regard God with the highest esteem, and ask what it is that He desires. He won't turn away from those who sincerely desire to do His Will.

In some cases, a high-risk woman may be able to reverse her condition. Many things, such as gestational diabetes and hypertension, can be corrected by a drastic change in diet and activity. Avoiding processed foods, white flour, sugar, and animal products will usually eliminate all disorders associated with diet, such as the above.

Other problems, such as the risk of uterine rupture due to a previous Cesarean, or multiple Cesareans, can again be helped by diet, and the avoidance of induction drugs. A diet that consists of mostly raw fruits and vegetables will renew and strengthen weakened systems of the body, while boosting the immune system.

Unfortunately, there are too many disorders to cover within the scope of this book. But with faith, common sense, and research, many–if not most, can be resolved or controlled. It is a matter of will, determination, and reliance on the Lord.

So after all is said and done, each woman needs to make the crucial decision of whom she is going to rely on: God, herself, or the medical establishment. She must handle her pregnancy, labor, and delivery wisely and faithfully. There are no obstacles that the Lord can't overcome, and He will meet each woman at her level of faith. Fear should not stand between a woman and a home-birth. If she has fear, she doesn't have faith, and without faith there is no hope either way.

Birth: A Closer Look

While laboring, the single most productive thing you can do

is to keep yourself moving. Every half hour or less, change position. This will help to move things along and encourage continual progress.

In addition to position change, keep yourself well-hydrated. Drink as much as possible and empty your bladder often. If you want to eat, by all means go ahead. It can only benefit your labor and the delivery ahead.

When the time has come for your baby to be born, you do not need someone to tell you when or how to push. Instead, it is a natural impulse. You should rely on your body and do as you feel inclined.

The first inclination may be mild or strong. You may feel rectal pressure, the need to pass a bowel movement, or the instant urge to bear down. As the desire strengthens, you will realize that the baby is coming. It does not go unnoticed.

The impulse to bear down may seem quite overwhelming. It is an involuntary action which you can try to resist, or work with. Most women find pleasure in working with it. It is, after all, the most active stage of labor. And your efforts will greatly aid in the delivery of your baby.

As the sensation strengthens, assume your birthing position. Be sure that you have chosen a safe and well-protected area. Semi-sitting on the bed or floor, squatting, being on all fours, or on a birthing stool are all very effective. Lying down, however, is the most unproductive because it hinders your pushing ability and does not utilize the force of gravity. This method is usually seen in hospitals, and is in the doctor's best interest, not the birthing mother's.

As the baby descends further down your birth canal, the pressure and urge to push become stronger. Go ahead and push as you see fit. If you wish, you can try and touch the top of your baby's head. It will be wet and soft. This softness is due to excess skin from the scalp being squeezed.

Most babies are born head first, but other presentations are possible. There are three main types of breech presentation. The *complete breech*, which is where the baby's knees are bent so that the baby's bottom and feet are the presenting parts. The *frank breech*, which is where the baby's bottom is the presenting part. And the *footling breech*, which is where one or both of the baby's feet are the presenting parts.

If you suspect a breech baby ahead of time, there are methods that can help to encourage the baby to turn around. The most common is known as the *breech tilt*. About three times per day, from thirty-two weeks gestation onwards, lie on the floor with your knees bent and prop up your hips about twelve inches or more. Remain in that position for about 15 minutes, or less if uncomfortable.

The most common position for a baby's head to be born in is called *occiput anterior* (OA). This is where the back of the baby's head (the occiput) points toward your front (anterior). The baby may also be in the less favorable positions which are *occiput transverse* (OT) and *occiput posterior* (OP). Occiput transverse is where the back of the baby's head points toward your side (transverse). Occiput posterior is where the back of the baby's head points toward your back (posterior). Sometimes an indication of an OP baby is extreme back pain during labor.

As the baby's head begins to emerge, it may seem like a game of hide-and-go-seek. When you push, the baby's head will become visible. As you retract your muscles, the head may disappear.

Soon enough, however, the baby's head will remain visible. As the largest part emerges, you will feel a burning sensation known as the rim or ring of fire. This description is accurate and speaks for itself. As this occurs, you may feel the urge to hold back. That is fine and a natural way of preventing tears.

As the head protrudes, it is a good idea for your husband or birthing partner to check the color of your perineum. White segments indicate that blood vessels are being constricted and you may tear. Now is the time to apply warm wash cloths with olive oil to help promote circulation and support the birth of your baby's head.

At this stage in labor, the contractions will be relentless and the birth of your baby is imminent. As soon as you catch your second wind, one vigorous push will deliver your baby's head. Then, the most difficult part is over. Congratulations!

Most likely, as stated before, your baby will be in the OA position. So as the head is born, your baby will be facing down. It will also be silent and still, which causes no need for concern. This is normal and he or she is still receiving oxygen through the umbilical cord.

If the umbilical cord is wrapped around your baby's neck, gently tuck your finger underneath the cord and slowly slide it over your baby's head. The umbilical cord is very elastic.

Within the next few pushes, the baby's body will rotate and swiftly slide out along with a gush of blood and fluid. A towel should be handy to help catch him or her, and caution should be taken. The baby will be quite slippery, and possibly covered in *vernix*, a white sticky substance that does not need to be wiped off.

At this point, your baby may begin to cry. If not, gently wipe off his or her face and use a nasal aspirator (or bulb syringe) to suck excess fluid from the nose and mouth. If the baby still does not cry or indicate breathing, refer to a professional for assistance and begin artificial respiration. It is wise to have an infant first-aid manual on hand which can direct your efforts.

If you are familiar with a certain method of artificial respiration, try that first. You may also do mouth-to-mouth resuscitation or the following.

1. Place one hand under the baby's shoulders and head.
2. Place the other hand under the baby's hips.
3. In a relaxed position beginning with the baby's body level, gently bend the baby's body by bringing the

shoulders closer toward the hips.
4. Straighten the baby's body back to the relaxed, level position.
5. Do this once every five seconds. This action helps to move air in and out of the lungs.

Once again, do not underestimate the power of prayer. It is reliable and effective, even when all else fails. If your baby is having difficulty breathing, command the devil to flee from you. In the Name of Jesus, command your baby to breathe.

Assuming that your baby is doing well, place him or her onto your belly or chest, skin to skin. This will promote mother/infant bonding and is a means to keep your baby warm. Cover the two of you in an old blanket to help retain heat.

The next step is to nurse your baby. You can assume the cradle hold and place your nipple in your baby's mouth, or allow the baby to wriggle their way up to your breast. Surprisingly, your newborn baby is capable of this. Nurse him or her as long as they want.

At delivery, the umbilical cord will be a bluish-purple and pulsating. Do not cut it! In doing so, you will instantly cut off your baby's air supply. Instead, wait for it to become thin and white. There is no rush, and some women leave it on until it naturally falls off.

When the cord is ready to be cut, tie a sterile shoe lace (or cord clamp) approximately six to twelve inches from the baby. Then tie a second shoe lace about one inch from that. With sharp scissors, cut between the ties.

As a midwife informed me, recent studies indicate that the umbilical cord does not require further care. There is no need for rubbing alcohol or other antibacterial agents. Instead, keep it clean and allow it to fall off on its own.

The delivery of the placenta will soon follow the baby's birth. It may occur anytime from a few moments to a couple of hours later. Whatever you do, do not tug on the cord. You may tear the placenta or hasten the separation from your uterus. Instead, wait for a contraction and the urge to push it out.

If the delivery of the placenta is prolonged and you are losing a sizeable amount of blood, you can take measures to trigger the delivery. Please note that bleeding often occurs as the placenta is naturally detaching. But if you are concerned, nursing the baby will aid in the delivery. You can also massage your uterus (through your belly), or use Angelica.

Once the placenta is ready to be delivered, one swift push will expel it. It usually isn't painful and does not require much effort. You should then place it in a bowl and examine it for completeness. You may look at a diagram to see what a placenta should look like, or simply make sure that no fleshy pieces appear to be missing.

After the delivery, you will probably feel sore and swollen in your vagina. Wet, frozen towels applied to the area will bring great relief as well as reduce the swelling. Caution should be taken when using the bathroom or showering.

In the beginning, your vagina may be too tender to touch. You can use a cup or a perinatal cleansing bottle of warm water to gently clean the area. When relieving yourself, it may sting if urine trickles onto your perineum. Try leaning forward slightly to encourage the urine to flow away from your tender area.

Once all is said and done, you may feel wonderful and able to go about your normal business. However, you must rest and take care of yourself. Nobody wants to deliver at home, naturally, and then end up in the emergency room for postpartum hemorrhaging. But this is a very real possibility if you underestimate the importance of rest. Bed rest should be a mandatory asset to your care.

In the face of chores piling up around you, bed rest may be difficult. However, remember that your well-being is important and needs to be taken seriously. So for at least two days, remain in bed.

You can use the help of your husband, friends, relatives, or a postpartum Doula. And remember, if your blood flow suddenly increases, this indicates that you are doing too much too soon. Relax and take it easy.

Within the first few days and weeks after the birth of your baby, he or she will have your hormones gradually draining from their system. But while the hormones are still active, they could cause your child to develop milk. This is normal. And even more alarming, but harmless, is to see your daughter pass blood-tinged discharge. This is temporary and poses no threat.

Some babies appear *jaundiced* when they are born, and in the days and even months following. This is characterized by their skin and the whites of their eyes appearing yellowish. It is due to elevated levels of bilirubin, a substance formed when red blood cells die. It is perfectly normal and no need for concern.

To aid in the reduction of jaundice, sun light is the safest and most productive route. In warmer weather, take your baby outside in a diaper, or naked, for a little bit each day. In cooler weather, turn up the heat and allow your diapered baby to spend some time near a sunny window.

The first weeks of your baby's life are the most exciting. They may also be the most worrisome, especially when odd things occur. It is perfectly natural to have concern for your child. Even the most confident and educated mother may panic from time to time.

The list of common newborn conditions is endless, for anything could occur. Some babies develop a yeast infection known as thrush, which is characterized by white spots in the mouth. Other babies may be born with a reddened blood vessel in their eye, often caused by the pressure exerted during birth. All babies have meconium, a dark, sticky bowel movement. And many babies develop dry scalp, known as cradle cap. Newborn hair loss isn't uncommon, and neither is acne. And most babies breathe irregularly, which is alarming to even the seasoned mother.

Fortunately, most newborn conditions are harmless and will resolve on their own. Research anything that you are unsure of, and look for natural remedies for symptoms that need to be treated. If concerned, consult a midwife, or a doctor who practices natural medicine.

Delivering a baby at home, unassisted, is truly a remarkable experience. Educate yourself, know what to expect, and know ways to resolve common and not-so-common situations. Fear often stems from a lack of knowledge, so research all that you don't understand. And again, remain in faith. Allow the Lord to show you this miraculous wonder, unadulterated.

Chapter Eight

A s I am writing these words, the final editing process of this book is already well-underway. However, as with life, surprises do occur, and it seems I've been blessed with another child.

You, my reader, are already familiar with the birth stories of my first two children, as well as the miscarriage of my third. Now I'd like to take you step by step, right along with me, through this pregnancy, labor, and delivery.

I plan to write in a journal format, updating every week or so, or more often if need be. I do this with the hope of giving you an intimate perspective into my thoughts, feelings, hopes, and fears.

The First Trimester

January 23, 2006
4 Weeks Pregnant

Although I was not experiencing any symptoms, I mysteriously awoke this morning with the strangest inkling to take a pregnancy test. So I did, and to my surprise, the faintest line appeared. I am pregnant.

Normally, I'd be shaking from head to toe with excitement, eager to tell the world. But I'm not. Instead, sadness, worry, and fear have swept over my body. It has been a year since my miscarriage, and a year hasn't been long enough to fade the memories that are clouding my mind. What if it happens again?

I am sure that the fear of a repeat miscarriage haunts every mother who has lived through the horrific event. I am also sure that I can either have faith or fear. Faith will carry my baby to full term. Fear may cause me to lose it. So it is time to build my faith. Pregnancy is supposed to be enjoyable, and I refuse to allow the destroyer to take that from me.

The date of my last menstrual period (LMP) is December 26th, 2005, which makes my estimated due date (EDD) October 2nd, 2006. My cycle has been regular since my miscarriage, but much longer. Because of this, my EDD may be inaccurate, and I will give myself two weeks leeway.

January 28th, 2006
4 Weeks Pregnant

For some reason, one positive pregnancy test is never enough for me. So I took another this morning, and I am definitely pregnant!

This time, when the second line appeared, I wasn't filled with anxiety. Instead, I felt excitement–the same excitement that overwhelmed me with each previous pregnancy. It was like a breath of fresh air, and a feeling that everything was going to be alright.

Fear had indeed kept me from being happy. I was afraid to rejoice. I was afraid to discuss baby names, to sort through maternity clothes, and to unpack newborn items. Most of all, I was afraid to love. Loving my baby would only make a repeat miscarriage more painful.

Early this morning, I awoke to pray, read my Bible, and

write down verses in my pregnancy organizer. I know that faith comes by hearing the Word of God, so the Word of God is what I need to hear. I wrote a few prayers to recite daily, one of which I have written below.

> *Dear Heavenly Father,*
>
> *Pregnancy is to be a joyous time, but mine is clouded with the memory of my past miscarriage. So I come to You, Lord, in the Name of Jesus, and I ask for Your protection. Your Word says that all good things come from You, which means that this child is a gift from above. I accept this gift wholeheartedly, and I refuse to let the devil take it away. My baby and I will only accept what comes from You, and we will reject all that comes from the devil. Your Word says that if I resist the devil, he will flee from me. I resist him completely, for he is not welcome in my life. Your Word also says that if I worship You, I will not be barren or miscarry. You have already healed me of barrenness, and I know that You will not let a miscarriage occur. I submit my body and my baby to You, Lord. I have faith that I will carry this child to full term and deliver a healthy baby–perfect in every way. Amen.*

I plan to continue this faith building throughout the entire pregnancy. I know that this faith will carry me through unscathed, and it is vital to my child's survival. This is not to say that the fear has completely disappeared. It is still there, but I am working it out. Building faith is a process, and as I fill my heart and my mind with the thoughts of God, fear will have nowhere to hide.

As for symptoms, I have experienced mild morning sickness, ligament pain, and a menstrual-type sensation. During each pregnancy, this menstrual-type sensation has always scared me, but I know that it does not indicate a miscarriage. A midwife once told me that I am feeling my uterus stretch, so I remind myself of that each time it occurs. A stretching uterus indicates a growing baby.

A growing baby isn't a dying baby.

January 30th, 2006
5 Weeks Pregnant

Now that the initial shock has faded a bit, the time has come to begin my prenatal care. Normally, I'd start by charting my nutrient intake, such as protein, calcium, and iron. But that isn't necessary this time. My diet is more complete than ever–consisting of raw, organic fruits and vegetables, just as the Lord intended. And because this is God's original diet for man, there is no room for improvement!

However, I am a creature of habit, and I will begin taking a high-quality prenatal vitamin and flaxseed oil, as well as continuing my barley grass supplement. I do this as a precaution to compensate for nutrient-deficient soil and other environmental factors.

In my pregnancy organizer, I will now be recording my weight on a daily basis, and my blood pressure weekly. I will also keep a checklist of reminders to take my barley grass supplement, prenatal vitamin, and flaxseed oil, as well as to pray daily for my unborn child.

Once I reach twenty-eight weeks, I will begin charting the baby's movements and practicing labor and birth preparation exercises. In addition, I will continue doing aerobics three times per week, but modified.

Yesterday I unpacked my maternity clothes, and they are now washed, dried, and in the closet. It seems a bit premature, I know, but I am so excited about being pregnant that I needed something productive to do with my nervous energy. I'll try to save the baby clothes for next week!

Every day, I have been reciting prayers for my unborn child. Along with these prayers, I have also been commanding my body and baby to function properly, and have listed one command below.

Body and Baby,

As I lay my hands on you, I command, in the Name of Jesus, that you function properly. Do not miscarry, do not threaten to miscarry, do not cramp, bleed, release water, or anything else detrimental to this pregnancy. I command you to be in perfect health, and to only deliver when the time is right. The devil has no authority over you. You are to submit only to God, so be well. Amen.

I have also been meditating on verses pertaining to pregnancy and miscarriage, repeating them aloud in order to build faith.

Exodus 23:25-26 Worship the Lord your God, and his blessing will be on your food and water. I will take away sickness from among you, and none will be barren or miscarry in your land. I will give you a full life span.

Deuteronomy 30:8-9 You will again obey the Lord and follow all his commands I am giving you today. Then the Lord your God will make you most prosperous in all the work of your hands and in the fruit of your womb . . .

I feel confident about this pregnancy. I really do. My husband and I talk about this child at every possible moment, and we are looking forward to the rest of the pregnancy and the delivery. Having children is such a wonderful blessing, and nothing compares to it.

January 31st, 2006
5 Weeks Pregnant

Nervous energy still has a hold on me, and I am battling the negative feelings that want to reign. Pregnancy always has milestones, such as feeling the baby kick for the very first time, but mine are different now. I look forward to passing the expected time for my menstrual cycle to begin. I anticipate making it through the seventh week of pregnancy, which was when my last miscarriage occurred. And I dream of the day the first trimester is over.

On a brighter note, my husband and I are considering baby names. Sometimes it is necessary to look into the future to stop worrying about the present. We both like David Gabriel and Marissa Rain. Even so, all names are still under consideration, simply because that is part of the fun of having a baby!

My husband says that he is going to throw me a baby shower this time. I had one with my first, and none with my second. To me, however, every single pregnancy should be celebrated. It is, after all, the miracle of life.

As for pregnancy symptoms, I have broken out with a few pimples. This is a first for me, and I welcome any sign that I can get. Let the morning sickness plague me, let my ligaments hurt every time I move too quickly, and let me break out with pimples if that's what it takes to help me realize that I am still pregnant and the baby is okay.

February 1st, 2006
5 Weeks Pregnant

Despite how bold I have tried to be, on the inside I was wallowing in fear. I'd worry about what I was feeling, and panic about what I wasn't. The dread grew thicker and thicker, like an impermeable fog, weighing on my heart at every waking moment.

This increasing sorrow caused me to realize that in the battle of faith versus fear, fear was taking the lead. My daily prayers and verse reading wasn't enough, for the fear was stubborn and deeply rooted. So I decided that it was time to step-up my faith building.

I have begun in the book of Matthew, and I read aloud a few chapters at a time, three times per day. I cannot describe the relief that this has brought. Not only am I building faith because faith comes by hearing the Word of God, but this action is drawing me nearer to God. I am now at peace, and even though some fear is still present, my faith is winning.

This is my second journal entry for today, but something so exciting has happened that I must share it with you. To begin, let me give you a little background.

As of now, nobody knows that I am pregnant, except for my husband and I. We've agreed to keep it a secret until more time has passed. We have also prayed for a prophetic word regarding this pregnancy, or anything that would give us peace of mind.

Today, my niece called me, and her words have answered my prayers. She said that she had dreamt about me for the past two nights, and felt the deep desire to tell me about her dreams.

In the first dream, she said that I was pregnant with another child. In the second dream, the child was already born–a boy. What a blessing!

When she spoke of her dreams, I felt tingles throughout my entire body. This was exactly the type of reassurance that I had hoped for, and precisely what I needed. I do feel that this is a Word from the Lord, and a sign that, not only is everything going to be okay, but we are going to be blessed with the son that we have dreamed of. Hallelujah!

February 6th, 2006
6 Weeks Pregnant

I've made it to my first milestone, and can breathe a little easier. Yesterday was the last possible day my menstrual cycle could have begun, and it didn't.

As for pregnancy symptoms, they cease to exist. I am not

experiencing morning sickness, tiredness, or any type of emotional upset. I thoroughly contribute these perks to following God's original diet for man–one full of raw fruits, vegetables, and whole grains.

Yesterday my husband and I unpacked the baby clothes, and sorted what we could and couldn't use. At the same time, we watched the home videos of my daughters when they were first born. Babies are precious, and I am beginning to feel that nine months is too long of a wait.

February 14th, 2006
7 Weeks Pregnant

Yesterday I reached my second milestone, and I feel even more relieved. I have now passed the exact day that I miscarried my last pregnancy. I feel wonderful, and everything is progressing smoothly.

For the past few days, I have been experiencing more pregnancy symptoms, but nothing major. I've been craving foods–specifically things I repeatedly see on television commercials. I've also been just a bit emotional and have had uneventful, vague bouts of nausea. I thank God for these small signs, for they reassure me that all is well.

The terror of miscarrying is still tucked in the back of my mind, but it isn't a prevailing thought. At times, the fear comes into focus, such as the moment before I wipe after using the bathroom, but it vanishes instantly. I am diligent in praying and studying my Bible, and I fully contribute my peace to the faith I have in the Lord.

February 20th, 2006
8 Weeks Pregnant

I gave in to a few pregnancy cravings, such as meatballs and pizza, and I am reaping the results. It triggered the onset of terrible morning sickness, which is fortunately tapering off since I've regained my self-control.

The pregnancy is progressing smoothly, and some days I feel so sure that everything is going to be okay. Then, in the blink of an eye, a sensation occurs that throws me into a brief mental panic. Only seconds pass before I regain my composure by reminding myself of the Lord's promises. Sometimes life just seems so fragile.

Recently, I've been putting a lot of thought into the baby's name. Today, in the book of Luke, I read how the angel, Gabriel, appeared to Elizabeth and Mary, telling them both that they would each have a son, whose names were to be John and Jesus. Just as my niece dreamed I would have a son, she also dreamed that his name was Michael. Is this a coincidence, or have I been given a name for my child-to-be? The answer I long to find.

March 6th, 2006
10 Weeks Pregnant

I make a point to post weekly, but as you may have noticed, there isn't an entry for week number nine. Last week was a very trying week–a week where my faith was put to the test.

My pregnancy cravings and aversions had been relentless, and I decided to make an exception to my mostly-vegan diet–dairy. I had a yogurt before lunch, fettuccine alfredo for dinner, and ice cream afterwards. As the day grew on, I felt worse and worse, and these dairy products triggered a severe ear infection.

I saw my homeopathic doctor the following morning, after suffering through a sleepless night with intense pain and pressure. I indeed had an ear infection, and was prescribed a natural remedy, as well as a prescription if the infection worsened over the weekend.

Despite my condition, and the rest I so desperately needed, Friday was a hectic day. I was having a big birthday party for my daughters the following evening, and most of the preparation needed to be done in advance because of the Sabbath. I spent much of the day tearful, tired, and cranky. There was so much to do, so little time, and nobody to help.

Early Friday evening, after hanging the last streamer, I felt an alarming gush of fluid. It was the same type of gush that occurred at the onset of my previous miscarriage, and dread swept over my already-weakened body.

Despite the situation, I refused to panic. The last time I panicked, I lost my baby. I didn't want that to happen again. The time had come to choose faith or fear, and I knew it. It was a subject that I had boldly written about, and now I needed to apply it to my very child's life.

I went to the bathroom and discovered that I had lost fluid, along with a lot of discharge. I felt sick inside, terrified really, for I couldn't believe that it was happening again.

Instead of crying and submitting to whatever was going to happen, I instantly turned to my Bible and prayer. I read everything that I could find on pregnancy, miscarriage, faith, and resisting the devil. I also called my messianic Rabbi to pray for me.

For the rest of the evening, I continually checked for more fluid loss, and even worse, blood. My uterus was tightening, a miscarriage seemed inevitable, but I refused to give up. I prayed and prayed, and spoke aloud the Word of God, specifically the verses that state that as a worshiper, I will not miscarry, and that as a tither, my vine won't cast its fruit before its time. I commanded the devil to flee from me, for my body to line itself up with the Word of God, and anything I could think of.

Friday night was the battle of my life. I couldn't sleep for more than thirty minutes at a time, my uterus was so tight that I'd arch my back to relieve the pressure, and I continually checked for more fluid or blood.

Throughout the night, at every waking moment, my mind was on the verge of panicking. The symptoms I was feeling, along with past experience, told me that I was losing my baby. The Word of God told me that I didn't have to. The negative thoughts were coming one after another, and I had to fight each one by reminding myself of God's promises. I had to have faith if I wanted my baby to live.

The night seemed never-ending, and morning found me exhausted and quite beat-up. My uterus was still tight and uncomfortable, and I did release more yellowish discharge, but the absence of blood brought my first victory.

Prior to the Sabbath service, my Rabbi, along with other gifted members of the congregation, took me aside and prayed for me. By this time, I was crying uncontrollably and I just wanted to give up. The thought of losing another baby was unbearable, and the uterine tightening hadn't eased at all. I was tired, discouraged, and hanging on to faith by a thread.

This small group of people prayed for me, and worked on binding the dominating spirits, such as fear, as well as breaking generational curses. Prophetic words were also spoken, and left me in awe. One woman knew that I was pregnant weeks ago, and also knew that it was a boy. Another woman envisioned crowns on my son's head, and yet another recognized him as a descendant of Aaron, meaning that he has Jewish roots. And still, another woman saw a fiery dart pressing against my uterus, for the devil was determined to take my baby away.

Afterwards, my husband and I went home, and I was dreading the party that was only hours away. I didn't feel that I could bear the burden of possibly losing my unborn child, as well as entertain a house full of cheerful guests who were oblivious to the ongoing trial.

Even so, the party went on as planned. I spent an hour or so praying beforehand, and commanding the devil to go elsewhere. It was almost like a pep-talk, for I desperately needed the encouragement to go on.

The party was wonderful for my girls, as well as the guests, even though I felt like I was dying inside. I had been battling fear for two days, along with an untreated ear infection, and my only desire was to collapse and give up. Behind my polite smile, I was suffering, for the events of the past two days were replaying in my mind.

During the party, an Uncle of mine placed his hands on my belly and prayed for me. I welcomed all the prayer that I could get. I knew that my son was so important that the devil had a great desire to take him away.

As the party ended, and the last guests left, I made the startling discovery that all uterine activity had ceased. This instantly brought about a great sense of relief, comfort, and victory. There was no blood, no more fluid, and no uterine tension. Even so, my heart still bled for my unborn child. I wondered if he had survived the harrowing events.

As of now, the uterine sensations come and go. They are never severe, and I like to think of them as aftershocks, since the earthquake is over. Tomorrow I am expecting the delivery of my fetal Doppler, and I hope to hear the reassuring sound of my unborn son's heart. The Lord has been with me, and He has fulfilled His Word which says that I do not have to miscarry. All I needed to do was trust in Him.

March 7th, 2006
10 Weeks Pregnant

It is early morning right now, and my fetal Doppler isn't expected to arrive until later. My mind and body are mostly at peace, but the devil seems to have found a new way to torment me. Days ago, I wouldn't have recognized this as the devil's doing, but as my own insecurity. Now, I know better.

Beforehand, I worried about what I was feeling—fluid loss and uterine tension. Now, I find myself concerned with the absence of pregnancy symptoms, specifically nausea. The devil is using this lack of symptoms, along with my miscarriage knowledge, to fool me into believing that my baby has already died, and that the bleeding will come later. Although this can happen, medically-speaking, I know that the devil is lying to me. I am quick to shun these thoughts from my mind, for the Word of God says that I do not have to miscarry.

Next, the devil is telling me that I am misinterpreting the Word of God–that the promise of a miscarriage-free pregnancy is only for the elect, or a precept of the Old Testament that is no longer valid. He is also telling me that there are exceptions to God's rule, and that I am the exception. Again, these are lies, and I refuse to be deceived. I am okay. My baby is okay. The Lord would not say that I don't have to miscarry if it weren't true.

Praise the Lord! My fetal Doppler arrived early this afternoon, and after only a minute of searching, I found my baby's heartbeat. What a blessing! I have now experienced another one of God's promises firsthand–the promise that as a worshiper and tither, I do not have to miscarry! Neither do you!

Based on the baby's location, which was midway between my pubic bone and navel, and the ease I had in detecting a strong heartbeat, I now feel confident that my EDD is accurate. It also appears that the placenta is attached to the right side of my uterus.

The sounds of my womb were intriguing–full of swishing, pulsating, and of course, the rapid gallop of my baby's heart. What joy it brings to listen to these comforting sounds in the privacy of my own home!

March 13th, 2005
11 Weeks Pregnant

Since my last post, I have not experienced any more miscarriage signs whatsoever. Thank God! I feel wonderful and everything is progressing smoothly. Most importantly, my baby is safe and sound.

March 20th, 2005
12 Weeks Pregnant

Today I have reached another milestone. I've made it through the first trimester, and the baby and I are doing great. I wouldn't expect anything less. I know what the Word says, and I've commanded my body to act accordingly. I am thankful to have a God who honors His Word.

Due to the events of the past few weeks, I had discontinued exercising. Now that the storm has passed, I'm back on track. I'll be doing aerobics three times per week, and I plan to begin labor and birth preparation exercises later on.

I listened to the baby's heartbeat today, and it was 161 BPM (beats per minute). As for me, my blood pressure is 107/67, and I've gained about three pounds total. All is well! The nausea has ceased, the tiredness is slowly disappearing, and the cravings are under control. I look forward to a blessed second and third trimester.

March 27th, 2006
13 Weeks Pregnant

It is a bit early, but I'm confident that I can feel the baby move within my belly. The sensation is subtle–a mere flutter–but unmistakable. This is a first for me, and can probably be contributed to two factors. First, I think that my previous pregnancies have left me with a heightened awareness of such things. And second, as a remnant of my miscarriage, I am quite obsessed with each and every sensation.

As early as it may be, I am already wearing maternity clothes. It isn't necessarily because I am showing, but rather because my regular clothes were putting uncomfortable pressure on my hardened uterus. I feel great, the baby is doing well, and my mind is at peace.

The Second Trimester

April 4th, 2006
14 Weeks Pregnant

My belly is even larger now, and the fact that I'm pregnant seems to be apparent to everyone. I can feel the baby move on occasion, but I look forward to the time when these movements are more easily detected. Each little flutter is a reminder that all is well.

At some moments, I feel so full of joy that I almost can't contain myself. Pregnancy is definitely a blessing, and the fact that spring has arrived only adds to my enthusiasm. My daughters and I have been enjoying picnic lunches beneath the deep blue sky, with puffy white clouds above, a warm breeze, and scattered pansies and daffodils. What a wonderful time to be expecting! Life is great!

April 17th, 2006
16 Weeks Pregnant

My pregnancy is passing by smoothly, leaving no need to update this journal so frequently. I'm great, the baby's great, and things couldn't be better! My blood pressure is lingering around a healthy 110/65, while the baby's heartbeat is equally as healthy, being around 150. As for weight, I've gained a little under 10 pounds.

I've discontinued my aerobic workouts, mostly due to the fear of over-doing it. As the stay-at-home mother of two little girls, daily life is a workout in itself.

This past weekend, I've had the pleasure of shopping for maternity clothes. My wardrobe is limited, but will do just fine over the next five months or so.

May 5th, 2006
18 Weeks Pregnant

Recently, I've been feeling a bit unlike myself. I'm normally self-confident and independent–especially when it comes to pregnancy, birth, and parenting. However, these strong traits of mine have been somewhat overshadowed by insecurities and the need for reassurance. I even went as far as visiting with a midwife just to have her opinion on the progress of my pregnancy. This is completely out of character for me, leaving me wondering if my faith needs some rebuilding.

Sometimes I think about how nice it would be to be cared for by another experienced woman, such as a midwife. I also think of how worrisome it can be to labor and birth alone. It seems less-stressful to have a birthing buddy–someone to encourage and watch over me, as well as ensure the safety of my unborn child.

This current thread of thoughts have left me feeling weak, guilty, and lacking in faith. I wonder if it is wrong to want to be cared for. I wonder why I feel such a need to be reassured.

To me, it seems that these emotions are being triggered by the memories of my past miscarriage, the possible complications of being Rh-, and the growing love that I have for my baby. Just like a child, I want someone to tell me that everything is going to be okay.

The baby is quite active now, and his movements are easily detected. Sometimes it feels like a little fish or snake squirming around, and at other times I feel a single thump.

Last week, while listening to his heartbeat, I almost thought I heard an additional heartbeat–not once, but twice. First, I found his heartbeat on the right side of my abdomen. It was in the mid 150's. A moment later, I heard a fainter heartbeat near the opposite side of my abdomen that registered in the 140's. Then, while listening to his strong heartbeat one last time, another noise–a beating-type noise, beat between his beats. It could have simply been him flipping around, or more likely, my own wishful thinking!

May 15th, 2006
20 Weeks Pregnant

Mid-pregnancy has arrived and everything is continuing to progress smoothly. The baby is highly active and his movements do not go about unnoticed. This acts as a constant reminder that all is well.

I have been experiencing more discomfort this time, including nausea, heartburn, indigestion, and constipation, as well as a severe allergy to dairy. Even so, I still love being pregnant. These ailments are a small price to pay for the creation of new life.

Fortunately, my insecurities of the past few weeks were fleeting. As a friend pointed out, my sudden need for reassurance was probably due to Mother's Day being near. This is my first pregnancy since my mother has passed, which has led to a myriad of mixed emotions–especially ones of loneliness and the realization that there is nobody to take care of me but me. I guess I was a motherless mother who needed to be mothered.

Although nothing can take the place of my mother, I did turn to the Lord for comfort. I had been quite distant from Him, and drawing near was a wise move. It helped me to rebuild my faith, and regain my confidence in Him, myself, and the body that He has so wonderfully made for me. It is strange how during the times we need God the most, we often go astray. I may have been lost, but now I'm found. Everything is going to be okay.

May 30th, 2006
22 Weeks Pregnant

Throughout this pregnancy, I've been anxious to know my baby's gender. I prayed for a son, my niece had a dream that I was pregnant with a son, and a woman at my synagogue said that I was going to have a son. All of these things lead me to believe that I am pregnant with a boy. Even so, I've been keeping my eyes open for a free or inexpensive ultrasound. Having a boy just seems too good to be true!

Well, I had an appointment today at a local women's center to have an ultrasound! Technically, the nurse who performed the ultrasound wasn't allowed to disclose the gender (due to insufficient training), but she could see my eagerness to know and was kind enough to at least search for boy parts.

During the beginning of my ultrasound session, the nurse and her assistant saw what appeared to be boy parts, but my baby was too active to really see. Then, toward the end of my session, a picture was taken that appears to show two legs with a little boy's "pee-pee" between them. The nurse seemed to know what it was, although she wasn't confident in her assessment, and definitely gave the impression that I am indeed pregnant with a son!

Besides the gender, my baby is in excellent health. He has a strong heart and quite a personality already. The ultrasound's measurements give me an EDD of October 8th, which is close enough to my original EDD of October 2nd. I just feel so blessed to have caught a glimpse of my precious baby.

David, as I'll call him now, is much more active than my other babies. He seems to be awake more than he is asleep, which makes me constantly aware of his presence. Every morning, like clockwork, he moves around. What a wonderful way to start the day! He continues to move on and off throughout the day, and always gives his Daddy a few good kicks before bed. I am thankful to have such an active child. It definitely relieves any miscarriage anxiety.

June 14th, 2006
24 Weeks Pregnant

Recently I've stumbled across something quite astounding

regarding the Rh factor. As you know, I am Rh negative, and as you may not know, most of my miscarriage fears revolve around this particular issue. It is frightening to think that, at any point, my body could begin attacking my unborn child–an attack that could easily lead to death.

Well, last year my husband was diagnosed with cancer. Although we submitted to one surgery to remove the cancerous mass, we rejected all other forms of treatment. This seemed foolish to most, but as believers, we knew that God had a better way–a way that He was just beginning to reveal to us.

Through months of research, I discovered that the majority of illnesses that affect humans, including cancer, are directly caused by diet. A diet full of animal products, processed foods, and sugar is what causes these illnesses. A diet lacking in raw fruits, vegetables, and whole grains is what allows these illnesses to reign. So we made a change–a drastic change.

I have now learned that these changes we had made will not only heal my husband's cancer and bring us all good health, but have the potential to take away my number one childbearing concern, which is my Rh status.

It is documented that quite a few women have switched their blood status from negative to positive by making the exact diet changes that the Lord had prompted my husband and I to make! I had always prayed that the Lord would just change my blood status, although I couldn't comprehend how He would do it. Maybe this is the way!

This newly-found information has encouraged me to adhere to my diet more strictly, as well as take additional measures to not only strengthen my body, but possibly switch my blood factor. I am in the process of designing a regimen for myself to follow that will not only strengthen my body to help prevent sensitization, but purify my blood to encourage a switch in status.

As for my baby, David, he is doing great. He is highly active and seems so much a part of the family already. His regular movements still bring reassurance, and I am thrilled that he is so active.

I've begun my first baby video this past week. I've recorded my ultrasound photos, a picture of myself at twenty-two weeks gestation, and the baby moving within my belly. I also plan to take some footage of my baby shower, my belly at later months, and the best part of all, his birth! I've never recorded my births before, so this will be really exciting to view afterwards. Of course, it will be for my eyes only!

June 27ᵗʰ, 2006
26 Weeks Pregnant

On occasion, I still find myself worrying, unnecessarily, about my baby. Is he moving too much? Is he not moving enough? What if the cord is wrapped around his neck?

These thoughts not only show a lack of faith, but an outright doubt in God and His abilities. God has already proven to me that He will sustain my pregnancy. First, He gave me His Word that says that I do not have to be barren or miscarry. Then, He followed through with His Word and healed me of infertility. And then, He saved my unborn child from the devil's attack. What more do I need?

My lack of faith reminds me of the faithlessness of the Israelites when God freed them from bondage in Egypt. God proved Himself time and time again, but it was never good enough. He brought plagues upon the Egyptians until they freed the Israelites. He parted the Red Sea for the Israelites, and then drowned the Egyptians in it. He provided manna for food, and He gave water from a rock. Even so, the Israelites still doubted Him. I do not want to do the same.

As for my baby, David, he is doing great. He is highly active and strong enough to shudder the entire king-size bed with one kick. He is also growing just as he should, although my weight gain has been fairly slow.

Each pregnancy is different, and this one is no exception. I get contractions each time I exert a moderate amount of energy, such as when I vacuum. They aren't the type of contractions that come and go, but simply the tightening of my uterus for a few minutes. My pubic bone also feels sore, which is a first for me. But all is well!

Chapter Nine

As unbelievable as it may seem (to me), I have finally reached the third trimester of my pregnancy. It's been a long and winding road, but the Lord has pulled me through unscathed. The end is in sight, and the time has come to plan for another God-assisted home-birth.

The Third Trimester

July 11th, 2006
28 Weeks Pregnant

Now that the third trimester is here, I will begin doing labor and delivery preparation exercises. I plan to do them on a daily basis, Monday through Friday, during a time I've designated as my "baby hour."

Preparation Exercises	Amount	Duration
Walking	1/4 mile	-----

Relaxation	-----	15 minutes
Squats	5	60 seconds each
Pelvic Rock	10	10 seconds each
Kegels	10	10-30 seconds each
Perineal Massage	-----	10 minutes

During my previous pregnancies, I didn't fully prepare my body for what was about to happen. Sure, I ate well, but that was the extent of my *physical* planning. Both labors were long and painful.

However, I've now realized that natural childbirth is *not* just intervention-free childbirth. Instead, natural childbirth is about planning and preparation. It is about encouraging your labor and delivery to progress swiftly and gently, *without* disrupting the course of nature. It is also about understanding the birth process thoroughly, instead of being taken captive by fear.

As for my pregnancy, everything is progressing smoothly. I feel great, and the baby is healthy, active, and measuring just as he should.

Surprisingly, I haven't gained any weight in nearly six weeks. This would normally be a cause for concern, but I've realized that since I'm not on an average diet, I shouldn't expect to have an average, text-book pregnancy. In a way, I'm on uncharted waters, and I will navigate as I go.

I've still been putting a lot of thought and prayer in to my Rh situation. I often ask that the Lord just change my blood from being negative to positive, but I now wonder if maybe I don't understand what I'm asking for.

From a medical standpoint, being O negative, like myself, is an advantage. O negative blood is considered the "universal" blood type, for it can be used in any person regardless of their blood type. What seems like a curse to me may be a blessing to others. Although I do not believe in the intake of blood, it is still an interesting thing to think about.

July 24th, 2006
30 Weeks Pregnant

Wow! It's hard to believe that I'm 30 weeks along already. I feel great, the baby is doing well, and I am enjoying how big my belly has become. Pregnancy is such a wonderful time, especially when it is not overshadowed by unnecessary worry and fear.

The weeks to come are going to be a bit busier than before. There's a baby on the way, which means that there are preparations to be made. Because of this, I've created what I call my "30 Week Plan," which outlines my intent for the last ten weeks of my pregnancy. (As you may have noticed by now, I thoroughly enjoy doing everything with lists, charts, and plans!) I encourage you to make a similar plan during this stage in your pregnancy.

30 Week Plan

Week of Gestation	Plan	Notes
30-31 Weeks & On	Continue prenatal care	Do as outlined in chapters 2, 3, and 11, including pregnancy tea, juice, supplements, and exercises.
32 Weeks & On	Begin planning/organizing labor and delivery comfort measures	I plan to use a birth ball, relaxing music, position changes, hydrotherapy, and general relaxation.
33 Weeks & On	Begin collecting birth supplies	Do as outlined in chap. 4.

34 Weeks & On	Begin perineal massage	Do as outlined in chap. 4.
35 Weeks & On	Begin Poly-Jean 5 Week Antenatal Formula	Take on a regular basis.
36 Weeks & On	Begin encouraging favorable fetal positioning	Avoid positions that encourage the baby to be OP.
37-40 Weeks & On	Make final preparations Strengthen faith	Get house in order and make final birth preparations.

As you can see in the above chart, I will begin taking the Poly-Jean 5 Week Antenatal Formula on a regular basis. For those of you who aren't familiar with it, it is an herbal combination that encourages an easier labor and delivery, more dilation before discomfort arises, and minimal postpartum bleeding, among other things. I have never used it before, but as I've said previously, I plan to be prepared this time. This supplement is highly recommended, and it is even more valuable to me as an Rh - mother.

Once I reach 36 weeks gestation, I will begin encouraging favorable fetal positioning. My last baby was born in the OP position (face up), which explains my long and difficult back labor. I don't want to go through that again!

Fortunately, there are things that I can do to help encourage this baby to be positioned more favorably. Most importantly, I should avoid positions that cause the baby to be OP, such as reclining, crossing my legs, and sleeping on my back. A baby's back is the heaviest part of its body and it will lay in whatever position gravity encourages it to. Because of this, I should spend more time squatting, sleeping on my side, and sitting upright. These actions will cause the baby's back to swing to my front, putting him right where I want him.

From now on, I am going to spend more time trying to figure out what position my baby is in. If he is positioned favorably, there are ways that I can encourage him to stay that way. If he needs to change position, I can encourage that too!

August 8th, 2006
32 Weeks Pregnant

Determining my baby's position has not been as difficult as I had imagined. The hand movements are gentle and bubbly, while the kicks are just that–strong kicks. Last night my baby was upright (head up), and I was actually able to watch him turn to being head-down. He jolted and misshaped my belly so much that it was truly reminiscent of an alien movie!

This Friday I'm having a baby shower, and I am so excited. I know that other people are supposed to plan the games and make the favors and such, but I love doing things like that. So, I am. As I've said before, each pregnancy should be celebrated. I feel blessed to know that my family and friends will be gathering to celebrate mine.

August 21st, 2006
34 Weeks Pregnant

My baby shower turned out to be better than I could have ever imagined. It was full of wonderful people, delicious foods, and fun games for everyone. I also ended up with many great gifts, including a beautiful wooden high chair and a co-sleeping bed. It was very touching to have my family and friends gather together in honor of my unborn baby. Memories mean a lot to me, and this baby shower has created memories to last a lifetime.

For the past two weeks, I've been experiencing frequent contractions. I'm assuming that they were caused by being very busy, as well as dehydration. I had been so preoccupied with my baby shower, a bit of redecorating, and my husband being on vacation, that my diet was easy to neglect. However, I'm back on track and the intense contractions have ceased.

My baby is still highly active, as usual, although he does have quiet days that tend to worry me. He appears to be head-down and I feel most of his kicks in my ribs. Every day I imagine what position he's in. I also picture what his little body looks like. I bet he's beautiful and perfect in every way.

This week I've been doing quite a bit of baby preparation. I've packed the diaper bag, washed blankets, set up the basinet, and organized labor and birth supplies. I even picked out my baby's very first outfit–all in blue, of course.

As usual, all of these actions have me feeling a bit reflective and sentimental. It is hard to believe that I am in the final stretch of my pregnancy and that the purpose for all of this preparation is about to arrive. One would think that this realization would make me nervous, but it doesn't. Instead, I feel content and at peace.

I have been diligent in doing my labor and birth preparation exercises, as well as drinking my pregnancy teas. Next week I will begin taking the Poly-Jean 5 Week Antenatal Formula. I feel fully prepared and eager to push another baby into this world.

August 29th, 2006
35 Weeks Pregnant

For a few weeks now, I've been experiencing a stretching/tearing type of sensation in the upper part of my abdomen. It's specifically located between the bottom of my ribs and the top of my uterus, slightly to the right side.

I do recall experiencing something similar in the last trimester of my previous pregnancy. It wasn't very bothersome, except for when I would lean over the kitchen sink to wash dishes. Fortunately, it never amounted to anything.

However, the sensation that I'm currently experiencing is

progressively becoming worse. It isn't too noticeable in the morning, but by late afternoon and early evening, I walk around hunched over in an attempt to relieve the strain. It definitely worsens when I spend a lot of time in the kitchen cooking, washing dishes, and doing anything else that causes me to lean over the counter.

Of course, there is a little part of me that wants to panic. I worry that this could be the beginning of uterine rupture, even though my rational side tells me that my uterus would rupture where my incision was, *not* the opposite end.

Another part of me worries that my placenta could be detaching prematurely, even though I have never felt my placentas detach in my previous births. In addition, my placenta seems to be much lower in my uterus.

So now I'm wondering about abdominal muscle separation, which is a more rational cause. Although it *usually* doesn't cause pain, *usually* doesn't mean *never*. Matter of fact, I've spoken to a couple of women who have suffered from painful cases of abdominal muscle separation. Their symptoms are quite similar to mine. I've also learned that this condition worsens with each consecutive pregnancy. It would make sense for it to have been mild with my last baby, and more intense with this one.

So, I did a simple test to see if my muscles were even separated. I laid on my back with my knees bent and my feet flat on the floor (sit-up position), and I raised the upper part of my body a little (like a mini sit-up). Sure enough, a bulge appeared right down the center of my belly, which clearly indicates that my muscles have separated. (For those of you who are interested, an indent would have appeared down the center of your belly if you had abdominal muscle separation in early pregnancy.)

Fortunately, abdominal muscle separation isn't anything serious. Once the baby is born, I can do exercises to correct it. This also goes to show that each pregnancy is different and you never really know what to expect.

September 5ᵗʰ, 2006
36 Weeks Pregnant

Due to the discomfort I've been experiencing in my upper abdomen, I've been trying to take it easy. Twice per day, I take a "time-out" where I relax in bed for about two hours to relieve the strain. During this time, I sip my afternoon cup of pregnancy tea, study my Bible, and pray. It is a very enjoyable time that I look forward to.

Besides my general prayers, I also pray for my pregnancy and the forthcoming labor, delivery, and postpartum period. I recite the following prayer daily.

Dear Heavenly Father,

First, I want to thank You for a blessed pregnancy. You have fulfilled Your Word within me, not only by healing me of infertility, but also by protecting the child within my womb. By Your grace, my days have been filled with contentment.

I ask, in the Name of Jesus, that You continue to bless my pregnancy. Allow my body to function properly without a single complication. Protect me and my unborn child from any adverse effects of my previous surgical delivery and my Rh status. Please keep us both healthy and whole.

I ask, in the Name of Jesus, that my labor begins when the time is right. Allow it to progress swiftly and gently. Allow me to remain calm, faithful, and of a sound mind and body.

I ask, in the Name of Jesus, that my baby be in the proper position for birth–head down and occiput anterior. Allow the umbilical cord to be of a proper length and the amniotic fluid to remain adequate and pure. Allow my baby to pass quickly and easily through my body, causing no damage to either of us. Please prevent me from tearing, hemorrhaging, or experiencing any complications whatsoever.

I ask, in the Name of Jesus, that my child be born when he is fully ready–not too soon or too late. Allow him to be healthy, alert, and perfect in every way possible. Allow him to have clear lungs and the ability to breathe with ease. Allow him to be of an ideal weight with no signs of jaundice.

I ask, in the Name of Jesus, that the placenta be delivered whole and in a timely manner. Please prevent me from hemorrhaging, as well as experiencing after-pains and any other complications. Instead, allow me to heal quickly and thoroughly.

I ask, in the Name of Jesus, that my baby is able to nurse effortlessly. Bless me with an abundant milk supply and protect me from any cracking or soreness. Please protect me from the baby blues and postpartum depression. Instead, allow me to be emotionally stable and able to adjust easily to my new baby.

As Your child, Lord, and as a worshiper and tither, I know that You will grant me the desires of my heart. You did not abandon me before, and I know that You will not abandon me ever. Please continue to fulfill Your Word in my life, and bless the rest of my pregnancy, as well as my labor, delivery, and postpartum period.

As the final weeks of my pregnancy are approaching, I will be especially diligent in building my faith and abiding by Your commandments. I want to please You, Lord, although I know that Your blessings have been given through grace. I am drawing near to You, and I have faith that everything will turn out just as it should. Amen.

I also recite the following commands daily, adding to them as the Lord leads.

Body,

I command you, in the Name of Jesus, to continue to be a safe and nourishing place for my baby to grow. Enable him to develop perfect in every way possible, just as the Lord intended. Do not gain too much weight, or too little. Do not deliver pre-maturely, or post-maturely. Do not detach the placenta before its time. Do not entangle the baby with the umbilical cord. Do not allow blood to pass between the baby and I, and do not become sensitized to positive blood. Do not cause me any pain during the pregnancy, labor, or delivery. Do not tear. Do not hemorrhage.

Instead, I command, in the Name of Jesus, for you to perform efficiently and flawlessly, delivering my baby in a timely manner without a single complication. I command that my uterus remain strong and intact. I command that my placenta remain healthy and firmly implanted until its due time to be expelled. When that time arrives, I command that it detaches gently and wholly and is delivered with ease. I command the umbilical cord to be of a proper length and to provide an abundant supply of air and nutrients to my baby until it is no longer needed. Amen.

Baby,

I command you, in the Name of Jesus, to continue to develop perfect in every way possible, from head to toe, inside and out, just as the Lord intended. Do not grow too slow, or too fast. Do not arrive too soon, or too late.

Instead, I command, in the Name of Jesus, for you to be born when you are due. You will align yourself in the proper position for birth, and you will come out swiftly and gently. You will be awake and alert with every system fully functioning. You will also be able to latch on effortlessly and sleep as a baby should. Amen.

Devil,

As for you, Devil, I do not come into agreement with anything that is not God's Will for my life. In the Name of Jesus, I bind any attacks that you have planned or that are already in progress. The Lord says that if I resist you, you will flee from me. I resist you with all of my might, so go, in the Name of Jesus. You are not welcome here. Amen.

Overall, my pregnancy is going well. My blood pressure has remained low, although it is gradually on the rise, and I've gained about twenty-five pounds in total. The weight is mostly in my belly, although my breasts have enlarged quite a bit as well.

As for my baby, his heart rate is in the 140's now, and he's still quite active. However, his activity is sporadic. Some days he feels like he's going to break out of my womb, while other days I have to pay attention to even notice him. This does worry me, but I've come to realize that this is just his personality.

September 19th, 2006
38 Weeks Pregnant

The abdominal discomfort I've been experiencing is still proving to be quite a nuisance. Although I initially contributed it to abdominal muscle separation, which may be partly at fault, I've now discovered that it is more likely a hernia.

This diagnosis was suggested by a midwife acquaintance of mine, and after some brief research, I couldn't agree with her more. Although there isn't much that I can do to ease the discomfort, at least my concerns have been laid to rest.

For those of you who are interested, my most prominent symptom has been a burning sensation in a particular spot between my ribs and navel, slightly to the right. It feels as though something beneath my skin is stretching or tearing. By no means is it a sharp pain, but instead, a dull, nagging sensation.

This sensation is more bearable during the morning hours, but gradually intensifies as the day wears on. The more time I spend on my feet, the worse it becomes. It is the most painful when I sneeze. Fortunately, however, I am not at all bothered by it when I sleep.

Last week, my baby went through a four-day phase where his activity level was greatly diminished. Of course, I still felt him move throughout the day, but it wasn't the vigorous movements that I had grown accustomed to. And although I tried to console myself by remembering that he does this on occasion, even my faith couldn't break through the dread that weighed on my heart.

Then suddenly, I awoke one morning to joyfully find the active baby that I had longed for. He was back to doing the twists and turns that misshaped my belly. He returned to his favorite hobby of kicking my tea cup when I rested it on the top of my belly. And he was back to kicking the bed during the night when I'm lying on my side. Oh how I missed him! And once again, I wonder if this phase was simply due to his positioning. Now I feel like all is right with the world!

I am thirty-eight weeks along now, which means that my baby can be born at any time. I would never ask for him to come too soon, but if it is the Lord's will, my heart desires for him to be born on September 26th, which is my wedding anniversary. My husband's birthday, which is October 15th, would be equally as sentimental. Or maybe my baby will pick a date all of his own.

I have been having contractions on occasion, and some have been quite intense. It is exciting, really, for I know that my body is warming up. I also know that one day soon these contractions will continue on, intensify, and aid in the birth of my baby. The simple thought that it could happen at any moment is really thrilling. I wonder where I'll be, what I'll be doing, and who will be with me.

The Labor and Delivery

October 2nd, 2006

On Tuesday, September 26th, around noon, I began having regular contractions. Although mild, they continued steadily throughout the evening. My husband and I eagerly watched their gradual progression, and we both felt confident that the time had finally come.

To our surprise, however, we were mistaken. The contractions simply tapered off, and despite our hopes to seem them resume during the night, they never did. It was our first bout of false labor, and the only thing it brought was disappointment.

I awoke on Thursday morning, the 28th of September, with more contractions. Due to the disappointment that had occurred just days before, I decided not to pay too much attention to them. They were more than likely "practice contractions," and nothing worth getting excited over.

However, around 11:45 a.m., as I was pulling laundry out of the dryer, I felt a gush. I immediately checked it out and found that I had lost a bit of amniotic fluid (a hind leak) and some mucus. Labor had definitely arrived, and my body was suddenly filled with nervous energy and excitement.

After calling my husband to tell him the good news, I spent the rest of the day preparing the house. I finished laundry, cleaned, and even went grocery shopping. The contractions were easily bearable, and I did as much as I possibly could.

As 6:00 p.m. came around, I began preparing dinner. The contractions had definitely increased in intensity, coming every five minutes or so, and lasting about forty-five seconds each. I'd pause during each one to concentrate on relaxing. Sometimes I'd squat, and at other times I'd rock forward, then back, on the birth ball. I also used this time to explain to my daughters, ages five and three, what was going on.

Later, my husband and I decided to go to bed as usual. The contractions weren't as intense when I was lying down, and after the busy day that I had, it was wise to at least try to get some rest.

I managed to sleep between contractions for a couple of hours. However, as midnight came, they weren't as easy to simply breathe through, so I decided to get up.

I spent the next hour pacing through my family room, while my husband and daughters slept soundly in the bedroom. I did one final prayer over my pregnancy, labor, and delivery, listened to classical music, and even enjoyed feeling my baby kick on occasion.

By 1:00 a.m. or so, which was now Friday, September 29th, my labor was rapidly progressing. The contractions were about a minute apart and lasting about forty-five seconds each. Each one was so intense that I needed to sit down. I tried squatting, but they hurt worse. I tried the birth ball, and they also hurt worse. I was the most comfortable sitting on my recliner, so that is what I did. I'd pace between contractions, and sit during them.

During each contraction, I'd concentrate on relaxing my entire body–focusing on my uterus. As each contraction escalated, I'd remind myself that the peak was near and that it wasn't going to get much worse. Then, as I'd reach the peak, I'd remind myself that the worst was here and it would be subsiding soon. I also continually reminded myself to focus *only* on the present contraction, and not the ones to come. I'd tell myself that I only had to deal with one contraction at a time.

At 2:45 a.m., during the peak of a contraction, my waters officially broke. It soaked my pajamas, the recliner, and even the floor. I was excited to have such an excellent sign that things were progressing, and even more excited that the amniotic fluid was clear. I then woke up my husband to help me clean up the mess.

From that point on, my labor became much worse. Each contraction seemed almost impossible to bear, and it took everything that I had in me to not panic. During the peaks, a part of me wanted to frantically jostle myself around to try and relieve–or at least distract myself from the pain. However, another part of me remembered the importance of remaining calm. I knew that I could have faith or fear. I also knew that I could labor calmly and in full control.

My husband saw the intensity of my labor, and thoughtfully suggested that I take a shower. I spent much of my previous labor in the shower, and it proved to be beneficial. So, I undressed and got in.

I stood under the hot, steamy water through a few contractions. I tried to squat. I tried to sit. I tried to lean on the wall. Nothing relieved the pain. Instead, the pain had worsened, and my only thought was to return to the comfort of my soft recliner. There, I felt safer. There, I felt more in control.

I spent the next few hours on the recliner. I was so tired that I no longer walked between contractions. Instead, I closed my eyes and enjoyed a few moments of peace. The contractions were less than a minute apart, and they were still lasting about forty-five seconds each. As the peaks would arrive, I'd press my palms into the seat of the recliner and slightly arch my back. To me, it seemed as if I was diverting the pain from my body into the recliner.

Around 6:30 a.m., as the sun was beginning to rise, I reached a point where I didn't think that I could possibly handle any more. I was exhausted–both mentally and physically. The pain was horrible and nothing seemed to make it any better. And, since the sun was rising, I knew that my daughters would be awake soon. I wondered how much longer the labor could possibly last, and even worse, I worried about what to do if the baby just didn't come.

During the entire labor, I was content to labor alone. Matter of fact, I preferred it. I didn't want any distractions, for it was important that I remained focused and calm. Even the gentle strokes of my husband's hand were a distraction, and I needed 100% of my attention to remain in control and relaxed.

However, as morning arrived, I reached a point where I didn't want to be alone anymore. I was tired, at my wits end, and now concerned because it seemed to be taking so long. So I woke up my husband.

As I was on the recliner, he sat by me. He encouraged me through each contraction, and comforted me between them. He also suggested that we pray together, so we did.

He asked the Lord for the baby be born within the next hour, but I interrupted him. I said that I couldn't possibly make it through another hour, and I asked that the Lord let my labor be over within the next twenty minutes. My husband agreed, and I think that I remember him laughing a bit, too.

My back was beginning to ache severely, so I decided to move across the room and onto the sofa. If I were to lie on my side, my husband could put pressure on my lower back during each contraction. I needed some sort of relief, even if only for a moment.

As I made my way across the room, I was hit with a severe contraction. I squatted at the side of the sofa, and the labor pain wreaked havoc on my body. I moaned, nearly in tears, waiting for it to be over.

The contraction peaked, and as it was dissipating, I began to grunt and push. Unlike my previous birth, I was not overcome by an unavoidable impulse to bear down. Instead, I just felt an inkling to push, and my body just did it.

As the contraction was over, I looked at my husband, smiled, and announced that this was it. The moment had arrived to push this baby into the world, and for the first time in hours, I felt optimistic. Both my husband and I didn't think that I was anywhere near this stage, and now here it was.

I climbed onto the sofa and ended up in a semi-sitting position. The next contraction came along, but I didn't instantly feel the desire to push. First, the contraction peaked, then, as it was fading, I began to grunt and push. However, my pushes didn't feel that efficient. I didn't feel like I was getting anywhere, and my husband couldn't see anything yet.

With the next few contractions, I pushed and pushed. For some reason, though, I didn't want to push, and I waited until I couldn't resist the urge any longer, then I'd push and push. My husband could see the head.

With my previous birth, each push brought about significant results. But this birth was different. Not only was the sensation to push much weaker, but each push only brought the baby a little bit further out.

Even so, only five minutes or so of pushing caused the baby to crown. As the baby crowned, I didn't feel any burning. I could tell that the baby had crowned, but I didn't feel the desire to push the baby out the rest of the way. Instead, I relaxed my muscles and tried to breathe. I expected for the baby to go back in slightly and the pressure to decrease, but it didn't. The baby stayed in the crowning position, not moving forward or backward. My husband encouraged me to push it out the rest of the way, but I felt, for some reason, that I needed to wait.

With the next contraction, I pushed and pushed and pushed. The baby's head was delivered. The worst was over.

As more contractions arrived, I pushed and pushed again. Nothing happened. I continued to push, but the baby's body wouldn't budge. So I gave one final push–a push strong enough to deliver the head–and the baby's body was born.

Within seconds, I heard a gurgled cry. My husband turned the baby onto its side and sucked fluid from within its cheek. He also gently aspirated the baby's nose. The baby continued to cry, and the baby's deep purple color began changing to a more lively red.

At that point, I asked what it was. My husband checked, and it was a boy! We finally had the son that we had dreamed of and prayed for. My husband covered our son, David Gabriel, and placed him on my belly. It was 7:43 a.m.

Although I am one to encourage immediate nursing, I felt very uneasy and decided to wait. My uterus was still contracting and I felt quite uncomfortable. I wasn't sure if it was time for the placenta to come or what.

A few minutes later, my husband cut the umbilical cord. He wrapped the baby in a blanket and took him from me. I felt that I needed to get up, and I wondered if the placenta was going to come. I felt weak and I trembled slightly. I also noticed a huge bulge within my belly on the right side, and it concerned me slightly. The rest of me seemed so deflated, except for this huge bulge. I worried that it could have been another baby.

I slid off of the side of the sofa and squatted over a basin. The urge to push swept over me, so I gently pushed. The placenta slid out easily and fell right into the container. Instantly, the bulge in my stomach disappeared. The contractions ceased, as well as the uneasy feeling. The placenta was the largest and most healthy placenta that I had ever seen.

Within about fifteen minutes, I was showered, dressed, in bed, and ready to nurse my baby. He was a beautiful baby, just like I had imagined. He was chunky, with lots of dark hair and short legs. His face looked just like his Daddy's.

At first, David had a difficult time latching on, although he had an easy time spitting up mucus. My first few attempts failed, but within a couple of hours, David was nursing like a pro.

My husband and I spent the rest of the morning in complete disbelief that we finally had a son. It was something so hoped for–so anticipated–and it finally happened. We finally had our David Gabriel.

David Gabriel was born at 7:43 a.m. on Friday, September 29th, 2006. He weighed a whopping ten pounds and was only nineteen inches long. He also had broad shoulders, which explains the delay in delivering them. Fortunately, he is perfect in every way possible.

Although the delivery was much longer than I would have liked, the Lord gave me nearly everything that I asked for. During the entire labor, I remained calm and in control. Everything progressed just as it should. The cord was of a perfect length. The placenta was delivered whole and with ease. I didn't tear or hemorrhage. I wasn't even sore or swollen afterwards. There were no complications whatsoever, and best of all, we now have a baby boy!

Postpartum

October 9th, 2006

Over a week has passed since the delivery of my baby boy, and I wanted to make one final journal entry. So many things happen during the first week postpartum, and I thought that I'd address a few of them.

David was born on a Friday morning, and by noon, he was nursing efficiently. Once he learned how to latch on and suck, that was all that he wanted to do. His every waking moment was spent nibbling on my breast.

Each time he latched on, I would experience after pains. My uterus would cramp, and it felt quite comparable to severe menstrual cramps. Although it was very uncomfortable, it was good to know that my uterus was doing what it was supposed to do. Through my belly, it felt hard and about the size of a grapefruit or softball.

I bled quite a bit during the first few hours postpartum, soaking about one perinatal pad per hour. However, after those initial hours, the bleeding decreased significantly. I did need to change my pad at least once during the night for the first couple of nights, but after that, I could make it through the night just fine.

During the actual delivery, David passed his first bowel movement. It came out with him. He then passed more meconium twice during the day.

On Saturday, my milk began to come in, although I didn't become engorged until Sunday morning. Then, my breasts were extremely hard and uncomfortable. David had a difficult time latching on, but he managed and seemed to love the overabundance of milk. I was very tender, and it hurt every time he latched on.

Saturday also brought about a bit of the baby blues. Some moments I felt very overwhelmed and concerned about how I'd manage my new responsibilities. I also felt discouraged. Instead of admiring my baby, I'd focus on the bleeding, the after pains, the engorgement and sore nipples, and the lack of sleep.

Then, as expected, I had optimistic moments. I'd feel great and able to take on the world. I'd admire my new baby, feel so grateful that nursing was going so well, and be in awe at how wonderful I felt. I never did tear, and I had no soreness whatsoever.

These wavering emotions seemed to last for about four days. I never cried, and I wasn't too bothered when I'd feel sad because I knew that it was temporary.

Around Sunday or Monday, David began having regular bowel movements. He'd go about three times during the day, and once or twice during the night.

By Tuesday, I can honestly say that I felt like myself again. The blood flow was minor, my milk production regulated, I was happy with my weight, and a part of me really felt like I had it so easy.

As Wednesday came around, David's umbilical cord came off. I never did put anything on it, and it dried up rather quickly. After it came off, however, I was a bit concerned about the appearance of his navel. It was a bit gooey looking and had a slight foul odor. So, to ease my mind, I began putting a bit of rubbing alcohol on it to help kill any bacteria. It worked well.

Overall, I couldn't have asked for a better labor, delivery, and postpartum period. I have been blessed beyond my greatest expectations. I am the happy mother of three beautiful children–children who are living testimonies of God's awesome power and love.

Chapter Ten

Poetry has been a part of my life for as long as I can remember. As a child, I wrote of the simple things in my world, such as clouds, trees, and animals. As a teen, my writing was centered around the whirling emotions of love and loss. And as an adult, my flare for writing poetry fizzled.

In no way has my work ever been comparable to that of the great poets. Instead, my writing is a therapeutic means for me to rationalize my thoughts and feelings. It is rhythmic, calming, and rewarding.

My most productive work is born through sorrow, although joy has produced fruit as well. Parenthood has brought many unexpected twists and turns, therefore reviving my desire to write.

The following poems reflect my innermost feelings–ones of barrenness, pregnancy, miscarriage, traumatic birth, and postpartum depression. In some ways, you may be able to relate, for emotions are a gift that we all share.

A Bridge Between Two Waters

Helplessly barren
Silence of fears
Hope long gone
Bittersweet tears
Prayers unanswered
Faith growing thin
Each month given
To lose or win
Soaring spirits
Flying high
To crumble away
So innocently die
A soul once rich
Now in the depths of despair
Still thanking God
For an unanswered prayer
A day may come
Ecstasy of life
A bridge between
Husband and wife

1999

Will I Have A Family?

Late by far
Half to be exact
Eager to know
Yet afraid of the fact
Wanting to be
Needing to see
Will I have
A family?

1999

Make-Believe

Years of trying to conceive
And left with the question of why
Why am I still barren?
God knows how hard I try
I'm too fearful to go to a doctor
For they may tell me that something is wrong
They may say that I'm infertile
And my attempts have been in vain all along
So for now I'll continue to try
To make myself believe
That it must just be bad timing
For one day I'm sure to conceive

2000

I've Been Blessed

I've been blessed by the Lord
For He has filled my barren womb
I smile from ear to ear
For I possess a life in bloom
He heard my aching prayer
And me–He did not deny
He forgave my many sins
For He's my Lord, my God, Most High
It is Him that I shall follow
With all my might I won't go astray
In Him my paths are straight
His Word I will obey
He's deserving of so much praise
With words I can't explain
My memory of this may fade a bit
But in Him I will remain

2001

Month One

A cell from your father
And from me–his wife
Became one as we in marriage
To begin your precious life
From those two that joined as one
New cells began to bloom
Dividing ever so rapidly
On their journey to my womb
The cells that are to be nourishment
Attach to my uterine wall
Connecting to you by a lifeline
For you are weak, fragile, and small
Before we know of your existence
Your heart begins to beat
Your face begins to form
'Though you are still so incomplete
And this, my child, is only
What happens in month one
We've a long, long way to go
Before God's work is done

2001

Our Family Will Be Complete

Some days
I feel as though
The time will never come
So overjoyed
And eager to test
The mother I've become
Yet other days
I feel as though
The time is running out
So overwhelmed
And taken by
Notions of fear and doubt
I can't wait to see
Your precious face
Or hear your heavenly cry
To hold you close
To comfort your fears
And sing you a lullaby
I anticipate
The very moment
When our eyes will meet
And the day
We'll take you home
For our family will be complete

2001

The Sun Will Never Shine

I had dreamt of this moment
For my entire life
Just the thought of hearing
Your newborn cry
Would bring tears to my eyes
I looked forward to the day we'd meet
When they'd place us skin to skin
I'd gaze into your innocent eyes
As you'd nurse and the bonding begins
Yet I was nauseous and I was drugged
With an uncontrollable shake
And you, my helpless baby
From my womb they would take
I don't remember when I first held you
Or the moment when our eyes met
All of those special firsts
I was sure to never forget
And now all is lost
And I don't feel that you are mine
The clouds above me will always be gray
And the sun will never shine

2001

Postpartum Depression

Our first nursing experience
Didn't include me
It was a bottle of sugar water
In the hospital nursery
The very day you were born
I didn't even get to hold you
I was drugged and unconscious
Pain was all I knew
I don't remember when I first held you
And now when you cry I want to hide
It doesn't feel like you're mine
It feels like my baby has died
I feel nothing but sorrow and emptiness
I'm in a nightmare that won't go away
I hope that I'll wake up very soon
For I can't make it another day

2001

I'm Drowning

What has been taken from me
Cannot be replaced
Not with time
Not with money
Nor with God and His grace
My wounds seem to worsen
As time passes by
The world goes on around me
But all I can do is cry
When I close my eyes I visualize
All that was done to me
Yet the moments I would have cherished
Are the ones that I can't see
I am trying so hard to move on with life
Now that you are here
But in my mind I'm drowning
With each and every tear

2001

All Is Lost

As an expecting mother
I expected so much
And I was willing to suffer
Without an allopathic crutch
Thirty-some hours I labored
I would have labored thirty more
But I was forced to deliver
The experience I now deplore
To others I seem well
In no one do I confide
When my baby was taken from me
All that I was had died
I was as strong as I could be
I gave my all at any cost
I'd do anything for my baby
But now all is lost

2001

Maternity Memories

My darling baby
Is down for a nap
I have time to organize
I am packing away
My maternity clothes
My favorite shirt
Is muffling my cries
The maroon fabric
Once clothed me
When I was glowing
And full of life
Until the day of delivery
When they slit me
With a knife

2001

A Crime Against Nature

You would never expect the sun to rise
An hour before it is due
For if you did–you would be a fool
And the world would ridicule you
You would never expect the tide to cease
Because your blanket is in its path
For the longer you'd wait–you'd be engulfed
By the ocean's natural wrath
Yet most things aren't as predictable
As the sun and the glorious sea
For nature itself has variables
And technology isn't the key
A perfect example is childbirth
And it is similar to nature's storms
There is a general sequence
And comparable ways the body performs
Yet you would never expect a woman
To labor according to time
For if you did you'd be called a doctor
Which to me is a punishable crime

2002

Empty Threats

The room was calm
And dimly lit
In my comfy pajamas
I could lay, stand, or sit
I would gently breathe
Slowly in, slowly out
With every contraction
There was no need to shout
My vitals were excellent
And my baby's were too
It was all so exciting
So pure and so true
I could eat, I could drink
I could do as I please
I labored with confidence
With dignity, with ease
Yet my waters were broken
For over a day
So I was taken to the hospital
And without delay
For my labor was active
Not much rest in between
And like I had dreaded
They began to intervene
I was told to change
Into a hospital gown
Into a lifeless rag
An abused hand-me-down
It was their way of saying
"You belong to us now"
For individuality
They do not allow

I was taken prisoner
As unjust as it may be
I was stripped of my rights
In this country we call free
They told me they had to induce
For the baby must be born
This is what had to be done
"For the baby," they sternly warn
They raped me of any dignity
And touched me as if I were their own
They exposed me without a care
And spoke in a threatening tone
Due to their lack of patience
The induction caused fetal distress
A life or death situation
For a C-section they now pressed
With fear for the life of my baby
I fought, but had to give in
It was a life or death situation
Or so I was told it had been
I then felt the urge to push
Yet they refused to acknowledge me
So engulfed in the thrill of a Cesarean
They ignored my heartfelt plea
I was strapped down to a table
With lights so blindingly bright
Confusion and chatter around me,
Too nauseous and drugged to fight
They ripped my baby out of me
Denying me my entitled role
Yet I am told I can still wear a bikini
'Though as a woman I'll never be whole

2002

No Loss

Something was taken from me
On that snowy March day
I was repeatedly raped
And brutally-I'd say
My body became the playing field
For the doctor's evil game
I was treated like a Jane Doe
My body–they chose to maim
It was a game of power and money
My dignity was the cost
Along with my life and my baby's
But to them it would have been no loss

2002

David 2*

The February snow is falling
A streetlight as my guide
I feel you move within my womb
My desires have not been denied
The clock has turned to four
You and I are silently awake
I feel so blessed for our time alone
A moment of prayer I shall take

Dearest Lord, I thank You
For my precious unborn son
Whom I do not deserve by deeds
But by Your grace it has been done
You have blessed me so abundantly
With the desires of my heart
Your Word is fulfilled within me
Let us never be set apart

David, first son of mine
The time is drawing near
For you to leave my sheltered womb
To the comfort of my arms out here
My God who has placed you within me
Will safely bring you out
Trust in Him for the rest of your life
With faith–not fear or doubt

2003

*This poem was written during my second pregnancy–a
pregnancy that ended with a baby girl, Cheyenne, not a David!*

Unborn Child of Mine

Child of mine–you've been a blessing
Bringing hope to my darkening day
To ease the crippling pain
Of my mother passing away
I have known of your existence
For such a very short time
I've had three whole weeks to love you
To dream of you, to shine
Yet my light returned to darkness
My hope suddenly changed to fear
Terror raged through my weakening limbs
As a gush of fluid appeared
So I laid in sorrow and agony
Emotions being turned and tossed
A labor worse than all others
The delivery of a baby lost
The grief is almost unbearable
Yet hope still wanders my mind
Baby, could you have survived this?
The answer I long to find
Although it appears that I have miscarried
That you are no longer here with me
I ache for a comforting sign
For my pregnancy to still be
Yet I don't want to clench hope falsely
And reality doesn't seem so kind
I want to remain in faith
Lord, please ease my mind

2005

Reminiscent Childbirth

I can't take it any longer
I thought, but wouldn't say
Enduring through the relentless pain
A baby on the way
Labor pains building
Like a raging storm at sea
Engulfing a tattered vessel
That vessel being me
A moment of tranquility
Then an overwhelming surge
Bearing down with all my might
Giving in to the unavoidable urge
Within a forceful gush of fluid
The momentous transition was made
My baby entered the world
No intervention, no aid
From daddy's arms to mama's belly
She latched on to my breast
Cord and placenta still in tact
Letting nature do the rest

2006

Postpartum Sorrow

My heart is full of sorrow
My mind has nowhere to run
With swollen eyes, so sleep deprived
I'm weeping from sun to sun
I can't fill the shoes that I used to
Too ashamed to let it show
Just plugging along as usual
With struggles that noone knows
Taking a day at a time seems impossible
For each hour is too much to bear
Imagining weeks is crippling
Carrying the burden alone is unfair
I'm haunted by haphazard emotions
Pregnancy hormones still wandering about
Desperately seeking a distraction
Some relief–a temporary way out
I'm a mother who needs to be mothered
Yet mine is no longer here
There's noone for me to turn to
I'm drowning in my very own tears

2006

Chapter Eleven

I have written this chapter specifically for the Rh negative mother. Being Rh negative myself, I know the challenges that this situation brings about, especially for the natural, biblically-obedient individual.

Since the creation of Rhogam, a vaccine for Rh negative women, little research has gone into blood status, leaving most mothers with two tough choices. First, they can accept the toxic injection, which is not only against the Bible, but life-threatening. Or, they can refuse the injection and risk never having another child again. Neither choice is pleasant, to say the least.

Fortunately, I've recently discovered that these aren't the only options. There are ways to strengthen the body, thus helping to prevent Rh complications. It may even be possible to switch from being negative-blooded to positive-blooded. And as always, you cannot underestimate the power of faith and prayer.

My Story

I discovered that I was Rh negative during the routine prenatal blood work I had with my first pregnancy. It came as a shock to me, for I assumed that if there were anything strange or rare about my blood, I would have known about it. However, a repeat screening confirmed that I was indeed Rh negative.

My initial reaction was to refuse the injection. It was unknown to me, and I worried what effects the toxicity would have on my unborn child. It was an issue that weighed heavily on my heart, and it took weeks to come to a conclusion.

Reluctantly, I agreed to accept it. My midwife, who I trusted at the time, insisted that it was perfectly safe for my baby and me. At that time, I was unaware that blood products were against the Bible, so on the basis of Rhogam being "perfectly safe," it seemed like the wise choice.

Considering that my natural birth ended in the surgical delivery of a positive-blooded baby, the injection may have been a wise choice after all. No sensitization occurred, and my childbearing future looked bright.

Then, about a year later, I became pregnant with my second child. By that time, I knew that accepting blood products was against the Bible. Rhogam was no longer an option. Instead, I was going to rely on the Lord.

My second birth was a gentle, unassisted home-birth. Afterwards, I did not have the baby's blood tested for status, or mine for antibodies. I decided that if I was going to rely on the Lord, I needed to rely on Him wholeheartedly.

My third pregnancy ended in an early miscarriage, and left me with the fear that I may have been sensitized from my previous birth. I had considered having my blood tested for antibodies, but soon realized that it had the potential of bringing about a serious dilemma.

If my blood were to test negative for antibodies, I would feel pressured into receiving the Rhogam injection to prevent sensitization. If my blood were to test positive for antibodies, then I'd have this dark cloud hanging over each subsequent pregnancy, making it difficult to remain in faith. So I decided not to test.

During the beginning of my fourth pregnancy, I had a

threatened miscarriage. I lost a sizeable amount of fluid, which was the exact way that my previous miscarriage began. However, I chose to rely on faith, and the Lord saved my unborn child.

As of now, I don't know if I have antibodies against positive blood or not. I also don't know the Rh status of my second child, or my third. What I do know is that the Lord sustained my pregnancy and there is nothing that He can't overcome. I also know that He is opening my eyes to see things that I have never seen before–things I'd like to share with you.

What is Rh Negative?

Simply stated, everybody has a blood type, either A, B, AB, or O. Everybody also has an Rh factor, which is either positive or negative. Most people are positive.

A person's blood factor does not have a major impact on their general well-being. However, it can affect pregnancy if an Rh *negative* woman is impregnated by an Rh *positive* man. Whether complications are plausible or not is all dependent upon which blood factor the baby inherits–the mother's or the father's.

An Rh negative baby is at no risk by an Rh negative mother, while an Rh positive baby is. If the baby's positive blood were to pass into the mother's blood stream, the mother may become sensitized to positive blood. What happens is that the mother's body recognizes the baby's blood as a foreign substance and creates antibodies to fight against it.

This scenario can have detrimental effects on the unborn child. The mother's body will attack the baby's blood, which can cause the mother to miscarry the child, even in late pregnancy, or deliver a baby with hemolytic disease. It is a scary situation, which is why most mothers turn to Rhogam.

Using Rhogam: The Risks

Rhogam isn't the cure-all that the medical establishment has made it out to be. It is not 100% effective, and some unborn babies will *die* within a week of exposure. Even worse, it is a blood product, which is not acceptable for God's people.

Rhogam contains the same toxic substances as vaccinations, such as thimerosol, which is a mercury derivative. Its use during pregnancy is very dangerous because mercury crosses the placental barrier within minutes of the injection. High levels of this toxic substance can cause autism, ADD, ADHD, learning disabilities, and death, just to name a few.

In addition, Rhogam is made with human blood. As with all human blood-products, it can contain a myriad of viruses, including AIDS and hepatitis. Even the latest medical advances cannot detect everything, and especially not diseases that are still unknown to mankind.

From the very beginning, God commanded us to avoid blood. As always, He had our best interests at heart. As humans, we cannot always foresee the consequences of our actions, despite how thorough we may try to be. That is why it is always wise to heed to our Creator's instruction.

Not Using Rhogam: The Risks

Most Rh negative women are told that if they refuse Rhogam, they will certainly become sensitized to positive blood. As a result, they will never be able to carry another child to full term, or at least not a healthy one.

However, there are a lot of "ifs" when it comes to Rh sensitization. A mother *may* become sensitized *if* her baby is positive-blooded, and *if* the baby's blood passes into the mother's blood stream, and *if* it is enough blood to trigger the creation of antibodies. As anyone can see, specific events must take place in order for sensitization to occur.

The passing of blood is much more likely to happen if the mother delivers in a hospital. Hospital births are by no means gentle, and any one of the numerous procedures can cause blood to mix. From an amniocentesis, to the common yanking of the umbilical cord, hospital intervention is the number one cause of Rh sensitization.

During a natural birth, however, the dangers of passing blood are significantly reduced. Special measures can be taken to avoid invasive procedures. For instance, the utmost caution should be used to not tug on the umbilical cord or hasten the expulsion of the placenta. Instead, things should be allowed to progress as nature dictates.

One interesting fact to take note of is this: During a typical hospital birth *without* the use of Rhogam, only about 15% of Rh negative women will become sensitized to their baby's blood. If only 15% will become sensitized in an invasive hospital birth, imagine how less likely sensitization is to occur during a natural birth. It is estimated to be a mere 2%.

As you can see, Rh sensitization is not as likely as the medical establishment claims, although it is undeniably a real possibility. You must weigh the risks, ask the Lord for guidance, and make the best possible choice.

Changing Rh Status

It is documented that there are a handful of women out there who began life with negative blood, but later *switched* to being positive-blooded. This phenomenon is deemed as an impossibility by the medical establishment. However, actual doctors discovered the switch in Rh status, *not* the mothers themselves. And, for the sake of clarity, these mothers were absolutely, without a doubt, negative-blooded to begin with.

This news is quite astounding for those of us who are also Rh negative. The idea of being able to change blood status is extraordinary, to say the least. But how did these women do it?

Surprisingly, each of these women had one remarkable thing in common. They each suffered from problematic pregnancies, and to strengthen their bodies, they all made drastic changes in their diets.

For the most part, these women eliminated all animal products, such as meat, dairy, and eggs. Instead, their diets heavily relied upon raw fruits and vegetables, whole grains, and pure water.

In addition, these women took further steps to purify their bodies, such as using herbs and colon cleansers. The herbs included angelica, bloodroot, blue cohosh, borage, capsicum, coriander, goldenseal, hawthorn berry, holy thistle, peppermint, periwinkle (which was the most common), sorrel, tansy, valerian, and vervain. These women also used wheat and other grasses, as well as ate foods that built blood, such as grape juice, molasses, and beets.

Once again, good health and longevity, even for an unborn child, can be achieved by returning to God's original diet for man–one of raw fruits and vegetables. This is a promising notion for those of us who are faced with the challenge of being Rh negative.

Preventing Sensitization

As stated in a previous chapter, diet is the foundation of optimal health. A healthy diet will produce a healthy pregnancy, and likewise, a healthy pregnancy will produce a healthy baby.

As a Rh negative mother, an excellent diet holds even more value for you. It will strengthen your entire body, including your uterus. A strong uterus is essential in preventing the mixing of maternal and fetal blood. Avoiding this potential catastrophe should be your top priority.

To strengthen your body, you must supply it with living

foods. The majority of what you consume should be in the form of raw, organic fruits and vegetables, as well as whole-grains and purified water. Avoid all animal products, processed foods, sugar, and all additives.

In addition, discontinue using fluoridated water and toothpaste. Fluoride interferes with the body's main protein that is used to attach the placenta to the uterus. Under no circumstances do you want to inhibit the proper attachment of the placenta, or encourage it to detach prematurely.

To complement your dietary efforts, citrus fruits, elder flower tea, and garlic will all aid in strengthening the placental attachment to the uterus.

Once your baby is born, there are additional measures that you can take to prevent or minimize sensitization. First and foremost, *do not* tug on the umbilical cord. And, of equal importance, give the umbilical cord adequate time to stop pulsating before cutting it.

If the delivery of the placenta is prolonged, *do not* massage your uterus to encourage the expulsion. This can cause unnecessary bleeding. Instead, wait until it is expelled naturally, or use herbs if necessary.

Really, the key to preventing sensitization lies within keeping your body as healthy as possible and having a gentle, non-invasive birth. Even more important is to rely on faith.

The Sensitized Mother

Years ago, before the creation of Rhogam, most Rh negative mothers would have one successful pregnancy followed by a string of miscarriages. Little was known about how to prevent sensitization, and nobody realized that the primary causes were malnutrition and invasive medical procedures.

Today, some women become sensitized before even

discovering that they are negative-blooded. This sensitization often occurs during a miscarriage, medical procedure, or wrongly-typed blood transfusion. Once sensitization has occurred, there is no use for Rhogam.

Fortunately, if a sensitized mother becomes pregnant with a negative-blooded baby, which is possible, there is absolutely no cause for concern. This baby is at no risk and will not further the mother's sensitization.

For the sensitized mother who is carrying a positive-blooded baby, certain risks do apply. The severity of these risks all depend upon the extent of her sensitization.

For instance, let's say that a mother becomes sensitized by an early miscarriage (which is unlikely). It is probable that the sensitization is limited, considering the small amount of fetal blood that would have been present at the time of the miscarriage. This limited sensitization would pose very few complications during this mother's subsequent pregnancies.

However, each positive-blooded baby that this mother carries will worsen the sensitization, thus posing more severe complications. On average, these complications will arise during her third or subsequent pregnancy of a positive-blooded baby.

For a mother who is highly sensitized to positive blood, her best choice would be to try to switch her blood factor, as described above. There is no specific scientific data that even proves that this can be done, but one cannot underestimate the effects of diet. I feel confident that the claims of the women who switched blood factors are indeed true.

Then, as with all things, there is faith. It really doesn't matter what complication a mother faces during pregnancy as long as she stands on the Word of God. God says that as worshipers and tithers, we do not have to miscarry. He also says that He will give us a full life span, which is a promise that includes our children–born or unborn. There are no exceptions.

Lifestyle Regimen for the Rh Negative Mother

As you've read thus far, there are steps that you can take as a Rh negative mother to decrease the likeliness of sensitization, limit the worsening of sensitization, and even alter your blood status. However, doing these things will require discipline, and possibly some major life changes.

I've devised the following five-step regimen for myself, as well as for you, my fellow Rh negative mother. This regimen will help us to strengthen and purify our bodies, purify and build our blood, and possibly alter our Rh status.

Step 1: Detoxification

The first step in strengthening and rebuilding your body, as well as cleansing your blood, is detoxification. This is a means to remove all of the toxins that have built up within you from the time you were in your own mother's womb. These toxins may have come from drugs and medications, pollution, household and personal care items, and yes, food. Most people underestimate the toxicity of what they eat.

The most effective means of detoxification is a water fast. However, as a pregnant woman, this is not a wise choice. Instead, you should simply eliminate *all* toxins from your diet. This includes animal products, packaged foods, sugars, white flour, non-organic produce, and the like. Avoid colorings, preservatives, flavor-enhancing agents, genetically-modified products, and caffeine.

In addition, remove as many toxins as possible from your home. These toxins can be found in laundry products, dish soap, bar soap, hair products, cleaning products, lotions, make-up, and similar items. Instead, replace these chemicals with the natural versions at your local natural food store.

Most importantly, drink water. Distilled water is the purest available, and you should drink it liberally. This will greatly aid in your body's ability to rid itself of toxic substances, as well as to regenerate.

For a bit of flavor in your water, add a squeeze of fresh lemon juice. Lemon juice is especially beneficial in the cleansing of the liver, which is the body's primary blood-filtering organ.

Freshly-extracted fruit juices are also beneficial when it comes to the detoxification process. Fruits are nature's cleansers, while vegetables are the builders. However, do not overuse fruit juices, for they do contain concentrated amounts of sugar.

The following is a concoction that I've recently created to aid in the detoxification process. I drink about two servings per week, and definitely no more than one serving per day. All of the fruits should be organic and run through a juicer.

Pregnancy Detox Juice

1 Orange, peeled *(rich in vitamin C, an antioxidant)*
1 Apple *(for sweetness)*
1/8 Lemon, with peel *(excellent in detoxification of liver)*
1 c. Red Seedless Grapes *(cleanses blood)*

Although there are detox teas available, I have yet to see one that is safe for pregnant or nursing women. It would be better for you to detox by eating pure foods and avoiding toxins, and save the more extreme measures for a later time.

The detoxification steps that I have listed above are meant to be a permanent part of your healthy lifestyle, whether pregnant or not. It is also suitable for your entire family.

Step 2: Health-Promoting Diet

Once you have detoxified your body, the next step is to keep it that way. This can be accomplished through the avoidance to toxic foods and substances, and maintained through a health-promoting diet.

A health-promoting diet is of the utmost importance to you because it will help strengthen your entire body–from head to toe–including your uterus. A strong uterus will be less likely to cause any complications during pregnancy, labor, and delivery. Even more important, it will be a solid ground for the placenta to attach to, making it less likely to prematurely separate or tear. Premature separation and tearing can both lead to sensitization.

Avoiding unhealthy foods is the first step to a health-promoting diet, but not the only one. What you *do* eat is of greater importance. At least 75% of the foods you consume should be in the form of organic, raw fruits and vegetables. Next to that, you may have whole-grains and other unprocessed foods.

Again, do not underestimate the importance of water. Replace all other beverages with water, and be sure to not mistake thirst for hunger.

As for supplementation, my highest recommendation is to take barley grass, or another grass. You will receive more vitamins, minerals, and amino acids from this source than any traditional vitamin and mineral supplement. This will help to replenish all of the nutrients that are depleted within your body.

To specifically strengthen your placental attachment to your uterus, try citrus fruits, elder flower tea, and garlic. All of these are beneficial during pregnancy.

Step 3: Health-Promoting Lifestyle

In addition to diet, rest and exercise are important factors. Both of these will help to strengthen and purify your body.

Be sure to allow yourself adequate time to sleep. If possible, nap whenever you are feeling tired. Even a fifteen-minute period of rest in a reclined position with your eyes closed will be beneficial.

As for exercise, walking is sufficient for a mother-in-waiting. Make a point to take a leisurely stroll each day, or take certain measures to increase your activity as you go about your daily business. For instance, park your car on the far side of the parking lot at the grocery store.

When possible, avoid hazards inside and outside of your home. Stay away from second-hand smoke, drive on less-traveled roads to avoid inhaling car exhaust, open windows when possible to allow fresh air to circulate through your home, filter your bathing water to avoid toxins that become airborne when the water is heated (in steam), and take any other measures, within reason, to protect yourself and your unborn child.

Step 4: Building and Purifying Blood

Building and purifying your blood go hand-in-hand. Both of these measures can be beneficial to all people, but especially to you as a Rh negative mother. For you, the main reasons to build and purify your blood are to strengthen your body, specifically your uterus to prevent premature separation and tears, and to possibly alter your blood status.

A health-promoting diet, as outlined above, is the single most important factor in the building and purifying of blood. A healthy diet will promote a healthy liver, and your liver's primary function is to filter your blood.

When working properly, your liver cleans about 99% of bacteria and other toxins from your blood. At all cost, you should avoid alcohol, refined sugars, and saturated fats. These three substances will hinder your liver's ability to function properly and optimally.

Vitamin C, an antioxidant, has also been shown to be very helpful in purifying the body in general. You can take it as a supplement, or simply eat a plentiful amount of foods that are rich in vitamin C.

And finally, herbs. Angelica, bloodroot, blue cohosh,

borage, capsicum, coriander, goldenseal, hawthorn berry, holy thistle, peppermint, periwinkle, sorrel, tansy, valerian, and vervain are all beneficial herbs that have been noted to not only build and purify blood, but also change Rh status as well.

There are also foods to help build and purify blood, such as beets, grape juice, and molasses. Do not consume too much grape juice or molasses, however, for they are both high in sugar.

The following is a tea that I've created to help support a healthy pregnancy and to aid in the blood purification process. It contains the classic pregnancy supporting herbs, which are rich in vitamins and minerals, as well as periwinkle for us Rh negative mothers. Steep one tablespoon of the herbal blend in boiled water, covered, for ten minutes. Drink at least one serving per day.

Pregnancy Tea

1 c. Periwinkle *(cleanses/rebuilds blood)*
1 c. Red Raspberry Leaves *(encourages optimal uterine function)*
1/4 c. Alfalfa *(especially rich in vitamins/minerals)*
1/4 c. Comfrey *(has pain-relieving properties)*
1/4 c. Dandelion Leaves *(nourishes/revitalizes liver, supports kidneys)*
1/4 c. Nettle Leaves *(supports kidneys, reduces hemorrhoids, nourishes circulatory system)*
1/4 c. Red Clover Leaves & Blossoms *(nourishes entire reproductive system)*

Also, most grasses, such as wheat grass and barley grass, are known for cleansing and rebuilding blood. If you are following my general prenatal care regimen (outlined in Chapter Two), then you should already be taking a barley grass supplement. If not, now is better than never!

Step 5: Gentle Birth

Lastly, most sensitization occurs during the birth itself. If possible, deliver at home or with a midwife. *Do not* pull on the umbilical cord. *Do not* cut it prematurely (when it is still pulsating). And *do not* take any additional measure to hasten the expulsion of the placenta. Instead, allow nature to take its course. This is what natural birth is all about.

Chapter Twelve

I have included this final chapter for prayers and confessions. Most believers realize the importance of prayer, but not so many realize the importance of confession.

When confessing, we are simply agreeing aloud with the Word of God. We are also building faith, because faith comes by hearing. Therefore, confessions must be said aloud, repeatedly, so that they become firmly established.

When reading this chapter, you can either read it in its entirety, or quickly browse to find what specifically pertains to you and your current situation. You can also modify the prayers and confessions to suit your needs.

Salvation

With this being a book for faith-filled women, I presume that my readers are indeed saved. However, some "believers" who feel that they are saved actually aren't, which is an eternal mistake. Simply being a good person will not earn a ticket to Heaven. Neither does the mere belief in God. These are both detrimental assumptions. Even the demons believe in God, as we see in the book of James.

James 2:19 You believe that there is one God. Good! Even the demons believe that–and shudder.

Salvation isn't difficult. God wants for all people to be saved, which is why He has given His one and only Son, Jesus. In order to be saved, we must follow three simple principles.

1. We must believe that there is only one God–our Heavenly Father –Creator of all.

2. We must believe that God gave His one and only son, Jesus, to die for our sins, and that God raised Jesus from the dead.

3. We must admit that we are sinners in need of forgiveness and ask to be forgiven.

Romans 10:9-10 That if you confess with your mouth, "Jesus is Lord," and believe in your heart that God raised him from the dead, you will be saved. For it is with your heart that you believe and are justified, and it is with your mouth that you confess and are saved.

Romans 10:13 . . . for, Everyone who calls on the name of the Lord will be saved.

So I offer a prayer for those of you who haven't accepted Jesus as your Lord and Savior, or for those of you who are unsure.

Dear Heavenly Father,

Your Word says that if I confess with my mouth, "Jesus is Lord," and believe in my heart that You raised Him from the dead, I will be saved. Your Word also says that everyone who calls on the Name of the Lord will be saved. Father, I call on Your Name and I confess that Jesus is Lord. I believe in my heart that You raised Him from the dead. I also confess that I am a sinner and I ask that You forgive me of my sins. From this day forward, I commit my life to You. In the Name of Jesus, I pray. Amen.

Infertility

Matthew 18:19-20 Again, I tell you that if two of you on earth agree about anything you ask for, it will be done for you by my Father in heaven. For where two or three come together in my name, there am I with them.

As mentioned in Chapter One, my husband and I stood on the above verse to overcome infertility in our own lives. The Lord does not show favoritism, and you and your husband can also stand on this verse. But you must be in agreement on what you are asking for.

During the early years of our marriage, my husband and I didn't openly pray together. When using this verse, we talked it over, agreed that we both wanted a baby, and agreed to pray about it–*separately*. It seems silly now, but the Lord still honored His Word. My point is this: Do not allow any apprehension to come between your desires to have a baby and actually conceiving.

Dear Heavenly Father,

Your Word says that if two of us on earth agree about anything we ask for, it will be done. Father, my husband and I are in complete agreement that we want a baby. We ask, in the Name of Jesus, that You heal the barrenness that has plagued our marriage and bless us with a child. Amen.

Matthew 7:7-8 Ask and it will be given to you; seek and you will find; knock and the door will be opened to you. For everyone who asks receives; he who seeks finds; and to him who knocks, the door will be opened.

Mark 9:23 . . . Everything is possible for him who believes.

Psalm 113:9 He settles the barren woman in her home as a happy mother of children.

Exodus 23:25-26 Worship the Lord your God, and his blessing will be on your food and water. I will take away sickness from among you, and none will miscarry or be barren in your land. I will give you a full life span.

Being faithful is a major part of overcoming infertility. Read your Bible and know what it says about having faith. Read it over and over so that it is deeply embedded within your heart, and let go of your fears. Fear works against faith. Fear is of the devil, and faith is of God. Be careful who you motivate.

Dear Heavenly Father,

Your Word says that if I ask, it will be given to me. It says that everything is possible for him who believes. It also says that if I worship You, I will not be barren. Father, I ask that You bless me with a child, and I have faith that it will be done. I believe in You, Lord. I also believe in Your Word. Just like Sarah, Rebekah, Leah, and Rachel, I want to be a happy mother of children. In the Name of Jesus, I pray. Amen.

You can also lay your hands on your abdomen and speak directly to your body. You can command your body to function according to God's Word. If you happen to know why you are unable to conceive, speak against it.

Body,

In the Name of Jesus, I command that you function properly. The Lord says that I do not have to be barren, and I command you to act accordingly. You must follow His Word, for you are under His authority. Amen.

Pregnancy

Pregnancy is often a susceptible time for many women, but it doesn't have to be. As a believer, you are under the authority of God. If you rely on Him, nothing can harm you. Commit your pregnancy to Him, commit your baby to Him, and rest in the knowledge that He is protecting you.

Dear Heavenly Father,

Thank You for the child in my womb. In the Name of Jesus, I ask that my body function properly. I ask that I carry this child to full term without complications. And I ask that this child develops perfectly, just as You intended. Amen.

Again, you can speak to your body. You can also speak directly to your baby. Speak to every part that you can think of, and speak against every concern and past problem. If you had a previous premature delivery, speak against it. Command that it does not happen again. If your baby had the umbilical cord wrapped around its neck, speak against it. If your children tend to be too large or too small, speak against it. If there are hereditary issues, speak against them. Speak against anything that concerns you, and have faith.

Body,

In the Name of Jesus, I command that you function properly. I command that you carry this child to full term without complications. And I command that this baby develops perfectly, just as the Lord intended. Do not gain too much weight, or too little. Do not deliver pre-maturely, or post-maturely. Do not detach the placenta before its time. Do not entangle the baby with the umbilical cord. You are under the authority of God, and you must submit to Him. Amen.

Baby,

In the Name of Jesus, I command that you develop properly. Be perfect from head to toe, inside and out, with every system fully functioning. Do not grow too slow. Do not grow too fast. Do not arrive too soon, or too late. You are under the authority of God, and I command that you submit to Him and His plan for your precious life. Amen.

Threatened Miscarriage

A miscarriage is every woman's worst nightmare, causing the first trimester to be a nervous waiting period. Oftentimes, the expectant couple will even delay the announcement of the pregnancy until this time has passed. But it doesn't have to be that way.

Exodus 23:25-26 Worship the Lord your God, and his blessing will be on your food and water. I will take sickness from among you, and none will miscarry or be barren in your land. I will give you a full life span.

As believers and worshipers, we *do not* have to miscarry. We are not of this world, and should not expect worldly things to happen to us. Our bodies and our babies are under the Lord's authority, and we can find peace in Him alone. It is again a matter of faith.

Dear Heavenly Father,

Your Word says that if I worship You, I will not miscarry. I do worship You. I have faith, Father, and I ask, in the Name of Jesus, that You protect my unborn child. This child is a gift from above, and I accept this gift wholeheartedly. Amen.

Body,

In the Name of Jesus, I command that you do not miscarry this child. The Lord does not permit for you to do this, and we are under His authority. I command that you carry this baby to full term, and I command for you to be a safe place for my baby to grow. Do not cramp, bleed, release water, or any other action that is detrimental to this pregnancy. When the time is right, I command that you go into labor, but no sooner. Amen.

James 4:7-8 Submit yourselves, then, to God. Resist the devil, and he will flee from you. Come near to God and he will come near to you . . .

In the face of a miscarriage, I know how difficult–even impossible–it seems to remain faithful. Your entire body is automatically gripped by fear and sorrow. However, you must remain in faith. Breathe. Relax. Meditate on the Lord's Word. Fear will only show the devil that he can continue to torment you. Faith will force him to flee from you. So draw near to God and He will protect you. It is not His intention for women to miscarry. Even the few times miscarriages have occurred in the Bible, they were all a direct result of sin, *not* a random act of nature.

Dear Heavenly Father,

It appears as though my body wants to miscarry. Your Word says that if I worship You, I will not miscarry. I stand on this Word, Lord. I have faith that You will protect me. I am drawing near to You Lord. Please comfort me and stop the devil from trying to take away my blessing. In the Name of Jesus, I pray. Amen.

Body,

In the Name of Jesus, I command that you stop showing signs of a miscarriage. Stop cramping. Stop bleeding. Stop leaking water. It is not time for this child to be born, and I command you to keep it safe until it is mature and ready. You are under the authority of God, and you are to submit to Him alone. Amen.

Vaginal Birth After Cesarean

For those of you who have had a previous Cesarean, you are probably well-aware of the future complications that *may* arise. Your uterus *may* rupture. You *may* hemorrhage. Even the medical establishment can't prevent the inevitable, but God can. Your faith can lead you a long way. And with the Lord as your companion, the odds are on your side (to say the least!).

Dear Heavenly Father,

My previous birth did not turn out as it should have, and the lives of my baby and I were endangered. But I choose to rely on You this time. Not a doctor. Not a midwife. Not myself. But You. I know that You are the Creator and are able to do anything. And I have faith that this child will enter this world just as it should–gently and naturally. I ask that my uterus remain strong and intact, and that my previous surgical delivery pose no threats for this pregnancy, labor, delivery, and postpartum period. In the Name of Jesus, I pray. Amen.

Uterus,

In the Name of Jesus, I command that you function properly. I command that you do not rupture. I command that you remain strong, fully functional, and intact. And I command that you contract appropriately, refrain from hemorrhaging, and release the placenta when the time is right. Amen.

Rh Negative Mothers

Leviticus 17:10-12 Any Israelite or alien living among them who eats any blood—I will set my face against that person who eats blood and will cut him off from his people. For the life of a creature is in the blood, and I have given it to you to make atonement for yourselves on the alter; it is the blood that makes atonement for one's life. Therefore I say to the Israelites, "None of you may eat blood, nor may an alien living among you eat blood."

Acts 15:20 Instead we should write to them, telling them to abstain from food polluted by idols, from sexual immorality, from the meat of strangled animals and from blood.

From a medical standpoint, being Rh negative is a home-birthing disadvantage. I can see why. From sensitization, to Rh disease, and even the possibility of your body attacking your unborn baby, it is scary.

As believers, however, we have something more powerful than modern medicine. We have our Lord and Creator, Who is omnipotent. There is nothing that He can't do. There is nothing that He can't handle. He knows your blood type, He knows the complications, and He can protect you and your unborn baby.

Dear Heavenly Father,

By no fault of my own, I am Rh negative. The complications that could arise during pregnancy are scary, but I choose to have faith and not fear. I choose to abstain from Rhogam, a blood product, because Your Word tells me to. Instead, I put my body and my baby in Your hands. Your abilities are unlimited, Father. And in the Name of Jesus, I ask that You protect my unborn child from any Rh complications. Amen.

Body,

In the Name of Jesus, I command that you do not harm my unborn baby. Do not allow blood to mix, and if antibodies are already present, eradicate them immediately. I command that my blood will pose no threat during this entire pregnancy, labor, delivery, and afterwards. You are under the Lord's authority and should act accordingly. Amen.

Delivery

Even after a successful pregnancy, the anticipation of the labor and delivery often brings apprehension to many mothers. As a society, we have been taught to be afraid. Childbirth is viewed as being excruciating, volatile, and dangerous.

1 Timothy 2:15 But women will be saved through childbearing–if they continue in faith, love and holiness with propriety.

However, Scripture tells us that we will be saved through

childbearing. Not only does this mean that we don't have to feel pain, but it also means that no harm will come to us. With God, the labor and delivery are nothing to fear.

Unfortunately, years of misinformation surrounding childbirth have been deeply rooted within us, making it difficult to view it in any other way. We need to retrain our thinking, and regain our faith in the bodies that the Lord has so wonderfully created for us. Childbirth is a natural, involuntary action. It begins when it's ready. It progresses as it sees fit. And it ends when it's ready.

Contractions are the most feared aspect of childbirth. However, a muscle contraction is nothing to be feared. It does not hurt when you contract the muscle in your arm, leg, and even stomach. It also doesn't have to hurt when your uterus contracts. What hurts is fear, which causes you to resist an involuntary action.

Building faith, as always, is the best remedy for labor and delivery fears. Have faith in the body that the Lord has given you. Have faith in His flawless creation of the female reproductive system. Remember that contractions do not have to be painful. Finally, practice relaxation so that you can fully focus on God during the intense moments.

Dear Heavenly Father,

I ask that this child be born when it is fully ready. Your Word says that I don't have to feel pain during childbirth, and I choose to stand on Your Word. I ask that I experience a short, painless labor and delivery. I ask that the baby be born on time, when it is fully due. I ask that it gently enters this world without complications. I ask that it is breathing, healthy, active, and that its body is fully functioning. I also ask that I don't tear, hemorrhage, or experience any problems or complications. In the Name of Jesus, I pray. Amen.

Body,

In the Name of Jesus, I command that you function properly. I command that you gently and swiftly deliver this baby when it is fully ready. I command that you cause me no pain. I also command that you heal quickly without complications. Amen.

Baby Dedication

1 Samuel 1:22 Hannah did not go. She said to her husband, "After the boy is weaned, I will take him and present him before the Lord, and he will live there always."

Luke 2:22 When the time of their purification according to the Law of Moses had been completed, Joseph and Mary took him to Jerusalem to present him to the Lord . . .

Matthew 19:13 Then little children were brought to Jesus for him to place his hands on them and pray for them . . .

Dedicating a baby is something that has been done for generations. It is a way to acknowledge that the baby is God's, given as a gift to you and your husband. It is also a way to commit that child's life to the Lord and to the Lord's service.

As you can see in 1 Samuel, Hannah dedicated her son to the Lord. In Luke, Mary and Joseph, the parents of Jesus, brought Him to Jerusalem to present Him to the Lord. Then, as Matthew shows, other parents brought their children to Jesus so that He could place His hands on them and pray for them.

You, too, can dedicate your baby to the Lord by simply stating so. You can also do it through a church or synagogue, or with a ceremony in your own home. If you wish, you can choose scriptural verses that you would like to apply to your child's life. I have created a sample baby dedication that you are welcome to use.

Dear Heavenly Father,

Just as Hannah presented Samuel, and Mary and Joseph presented Jesus, I/we come on this very day to present my/our child, _____, before You. You are the Creator, and this child is the work of Your hands. You knit him/her together in the womb. Your eyes saw his/her unformed body. And You delivered him/her into my/our loving arms. From this day forward, I/we dedicate my/our child, _____, to You. I/we ask that You bless him/her and keep him/her from harms way. And I/we ask that he/she serves You all the days of his/her life.

As a parent, Lord, I/we promise to train him/her in the way that he/she should go. And I/we know that when he/she is old, he/she will not turn from it. I/we promise to teach him/her Your commandments. I/we promise to discipline him/her according to Your Word.

Thank You, Father, for choosing me/us to be the steward/s of this blessing. May You bless me/us with the wisdom and patience to raise him/her as You desire. And may You bless my/our child, _____, with prosperity in every aspect of his/her life. In the Name of Jesus, I/we pray. Amen.

Final Thoughts

My desire in writing this book was to help guide you in the right direction. Sometimes it is difficult to see through the world's corruption and even the most diligent of us stumble. But the Lord has a way of doing everything, and His way is always the best. His way is the natural way.

John 15:18 If the world hates you, keep in mind that it hated me first. If you belonged to the world, it would love you as its own. As it is, you do not belong to the world, but I have chosen you out of the world. That is why the world hates you.

As believers, we are in this world, but are not of this world. The world hated our precious Savior so much that it sentenced Him to a torturous death. As His followers, the world will also hate us and our ways. But we need to remain strong in faith and persevere.

The world, today, is a truly scary place. Right is wrong and wrong is right. Those of us who care enough about our children to go against the flow are usually labeled as unfit parents. And I guess, in a way, we are unfit.

We don't fit into a society that rapes and mutilates women's bodies in the name of childbirth. We also don't fit into a society that subjects themselves to deadly and unnecessary medical procedures. We don't administer our children with fatal vaccinations, nor do we feed them the concoction they call formula. We don't entrust our children to daycare and morally-corrupt school systems. We don't honor pagan rituals in the Name of God. Simply stated, we don't accept the modern way of life to be *the* way of life.

Instead, we want to raise our children by the Lord's standards, not the world's. We want to teach our children what He commands, not that of the so-called professionals and the media. Above all, we want to do His Will, even if it isn't common or socially-acceptable.

As a society, we have been fooled into believing many fallacies that are in direct violation of the Bible. As faith-filled women, we need to help empower other women to restore the God-honoring lives that have been taken from us. We also need to stop submitting ourselves and our families to the world. We are God's children and are under His authority.

I hope that I have helped you in some small way. I feel blessed that the Lord has opened my eyes to see my duty as a faith-filled woman. I wouldn't have it any other way.

Regardless of your situation, the Lord can do miraculous things. Even in the midst of the impossible, He is a ray of light that can penetrate your darkest moment. Have faith. Trust in Him. Study His Word. And joyfully accept all of the blessings that come your way. Even more, rest in the peace that comes by simply knowing Him. May the Lord be with you and may you desire to know His heart.

About the Author

Lyra M. Camacho is a devoted wife and stay-at-home mother. Her interests include writing, singing, playing piano, and photography. She strongly supports natural birth, breast-feeding, vaccination education, and home-schooling. In addition, she is a proud part of the Messianic Jewish movement.

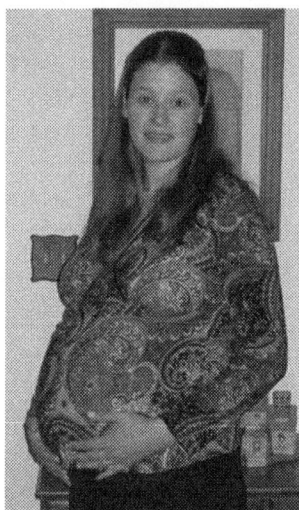

Currently, Lyra M. Camacho resides in the beautiful state of Pennsylvania with her husband of nine years, Joel, and three children, Natalia, Cheyenne, and David. She thoroughly enjoys being a wife and mother and aspires to help other women realize the profound importance of such a role.

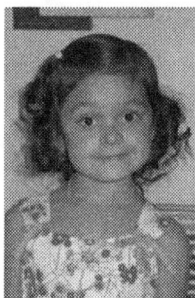

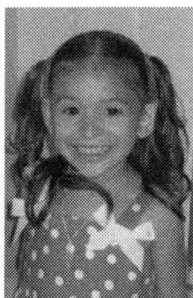

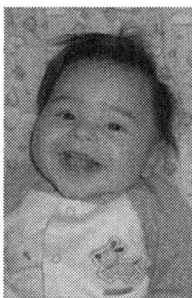

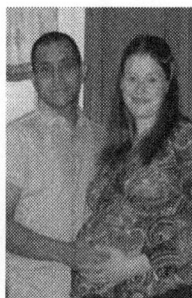

Bibliography

Block, Polly
Polly's Birth Book: Obstetrics for the Home
Hearthspun Publishing: American Fork, Utah, 1984

Campbell, Nancy
Be Fruitful & Multiply
Vision Forum Ministries: San Antonio, Texas, 2003

Cohen-Wainer, Nancy, and Estner, Lois J.
Silent Knife
Bergin & Garvey Publishers: Westport, Connecticut, 1983

Cutler, Ellen, M.D.
The Food Allergy Cure
Harmony Books: New York, New York, 2001

Davis, Elizabeth
Heart & Hands
Elizabeth Davis, 1997

Douglas, Ann
The Mother of All Pregnancy Books
Wiley Publishing: New York, New York, 2002

Karp, Harvey, M.D.
The Happiest Baby on the Block
Bantam Dell–A Division of Random House, Inc.: New York,
New York, 2002

Malkmus, George H.
God's Way to Ultimate Health
Hallelujah Acres Publishing: Shelby, North Carolina, 1995

Mize, Jackie
Supernatural Childbirth
Harrison House, Inc.: Tulsa, Oklahoma, 1993

Mueser, Anne Marie, Ed.D, and Verrilli, George E., M.D.,
F.A.C.O.G.
While Waiting
St. Martin's Press, Inc.: New York, New York, 1989

Neustaedter, Randall, O.M.D.
The Vaccine Guide
North Atlantic Books and Homeopathic Educational Services:
Berkeley, California, 1996

Simpkin, Penny, P.T.
The Birth Partner
The Harvard Common Press: Boston, Massachusetts, 2001

White, Gregory J., M.D.
Emergency Childbirth
Napsac Reproductions: Marble Hill, Missouri, 1998